W9-BNC-934

What is it like to be a nursing-home resident?

What preparations should you and your loved ones make for moving into a nursing home or retirement community?

In this unique book the "Robert Schuller of the nursing home set" shares the advice and humor of almost a decade of life in a nursing home. It *is* possible to live a rich and rewarding life in a nursing home—if you live it the way Opal Hutchins Sollenberger has!

I Chose to Live in a Nursing Home

OPAL HUTCHINS SOLLENBERGER

FIRST EDITION

ISBN 0-89191-242-8
LC 79-57521

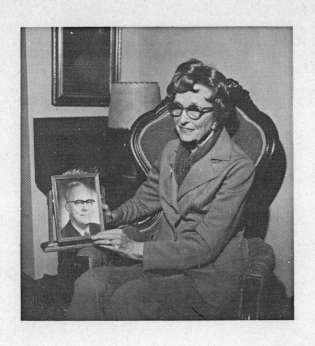

In memory of
Laurel
My almost-perfect husband for fifty-four years.

This book could not have been
written without the faith he
always had in me. His spirit
lingers with me still and
gives me courage to forge on
without his physical presence.

Contents

Foreword

Entering a nursing home can be a traumatic experience. Some elderly persons face the prospect with dread, others with apathetic resignation, and some with hostile resistance. There are also, of course, many who come to these final years with a continuingly positive attitude toward life.

Such a happy, exuberant lady—and astute observer of human nature—is Opal Hutchins Sollenberger, whose book is humorous, instructive, and inspirational. For her, every day is like entering an elevator and deciding to push the up button rather than the down one. She rejoices in the possessions—wisely brought from her home—that grace her room and keep her memories freshly alive. Living at Valley is a daily adventure of the spirit for her, a challenge to remain hopeful, an opportunity to bring cheer to everyone she sees in the daily round of activities. Through the pages of her book you will meet a charming companion whose wisdom and genial wit will engage you through several hours of profitable reading.

The considerations Mrs. Sollenberger suggests should be part of the planning that precedes the choice of a nursing home. They will be helpful to many who are preparing to make the choice themselves, or to those relatives who are making such decisions for them

While many books have been written about nursing homes by outside observers, this book is unique because it details the personal experiences of one who has been a resident of such a home since 1971. She has found contentment in living at Valley partly because she brought with her a rich treasure of inner resources, and partly because she and her husband, Laurel, planned carefully before residence in a nursing home became necessary. But fundamental to her joyous response to life at eighty-three is her steady assurance of God's presence and of his good purposes for her life.

Several friends of mine who have recently been faced with the choice of a nursing home for elderly parents concur with the suggestions presented by the author. Most nursing homes operate under state law. One should discover, therefore, if the institution is properly licensed. Does the chief administrator have the proper qualifications and experience for his position? Do the nurses and nurse's aides have the proper credentials for the services they perform? Is the institution financially solvent; is the accounting program periodically audited; is an annual financial statement available for examination? Are the immediate and long-range costs made clear—the entrance endowment fee, monthly residence costs, and any escalation cost clauses intended to keep pace with inflation?

Homes may differ greatly in their general attractiveness and cheerful tone. Some have been clearly planned with aesthetic grace and charm. Others may be extremely plain, lacking color and warmth.

The dining room, lounges, recreational and craft centers should be examined carefully for accessibility, comfort, and safety. Christians will want to know if there is a chaplain and a pleasant place for worship

Family members who are seeing loved ones through these years want nursing-home personnel who care and are affectionate. A single visit to a prospective home may not be enough to fully reveal this kind of concern, or lack of it. To feel assured that there is a sense of compassion for the residents, a conference with a family who have had experience with the home is helpful. Two or three favorable opinions are likely to give one a sense of confidence in the institution.

Opal Sollenberger's cheerful and optimistic account of her nursing-home experiences provides a new perspective on the possibilities for a rich and satisfying life in the summit years and will be a source of encouragement and help to many.

–PAUL M. BECHTEL
Professor Emeritus of English
Wheaton College
Wheaton, Illinois

Preface

The nursing home I live in (notice I said "live," not "stay") will never reach newspaper headlines for gross neglect or cruel treatment. And I'm equally convinced there are hundreds of other nursing homes like mine that are doing an honest job of trying to make our senior years as pleasant as possible.

Not all nursing homes are as ogreish as people think they are. Many seek to meet the physical, spiritual, mental, and emotional needs of the residents.

That is why I have chosen to write about nursing-home living from a positive viewpoint. I am tired of reading books that tell only what is wrong with nursing homes, without any commendation. A more balanced perspective is badly needed.

At the age of seventy-five I moved to Valley Nursing Home.* I have lived here happily since 1971. I think of Valley less as an institution and more as an excellent motel. Help is available at the ring of a buzzer, nurses and aides are concerned about me, and I have a beautiful apartment to live in. Whenever I need it, it converts instantly into a good nursing facility.

But it didn't just "happen" that way. It wasn't luck. It took careful preparation and planning. That's what makes the difference between the person who thoroughly enjoys life in a nursing home or retirement community and the person who is miserable, just waiting for death to occur.

Through the years I have observed that those who have the most difficult time adjusting to nursing-home living are those forced to move to unfamiliar places without having any say in the matter. That's why my husband and I evaluated nursing homes and their alternatives while we were still healthy and agile.

Because we started looking long before we had to, we were able to choose carefully and well. Because we had checked out the alternatives, we knew exactly what we wanted, so when my husband died I knew just what to do.

Most people don't know how to go about selecting the "right" nursing home. Many others would like to know how to make life pleasant for their parents or friends already living in such a facility. And almost everyone has misconceptions about a way of life that will touch almost all of us sometime after middle age. (See Appendix I.)

I wrote this book to answer some of those questions. The story of how and why I chose Valley should help others in their search for a good nursing home. It is my hope that when the reading is over and informed family members have discussed the alternatives with their aging loved ones, any fear, guilt, or doubt about the possibility of finding a good nursing home will be gone.

*The names of the nursing home, staff, and residents have been changed to protect their privacy.

14

I

"How Can You Stand It Here, Opal?"

I don't suppose they even had time to notice the two weathervane bird feeders and bird bath just outside my windows. Or the binoculars and guidebooks I used to enjoy the birds. They were only "passing through" and stayed not more than half an hour. These friendly acquaintances, whose last name I don't even remember, arrived at the Valley Nursing Home at one of the most inopportune times possible.

My husband, Laurel, and I had met them for the first time some years ago at the Everglades National Park in Florida. That year we spent several winter weeks there in our custom-made Airstream travel trailers. As is often the case, we met "on the trail" again a number of times.

After his retirement, Laurel and I traveled happily

about half the year for twelve years. The other half we spent at our Dutch Colonial house, "Glenside," its gardens surrounded on both sides with glens and brooks. We enjoyed growing flowers and vegetables, entertaining, picnicking, eating outdoors at every opportunity, attending theater performances, pursuing our many hobbies, and just celebrating life.

Bob and Ruth had stopped at Glenside once and seen how we lived. Knowing how happy we had been, they were curious as to how I felt about living in a nursing home. That's why they stopped to see me.

How were they to know that ninety-four-year-old Walker, sitting on a lawn chair in the entrance way, was wearing only one glove because he has an artificial arm and hand? He tried to talk to them cleverly and wittily. How were they to understand, in this brief moment, that he was almost totally deaf, always intensely friendly, and oh, so lonely?

When they were inside the foyer, they were greeted by a sweet little old lady who has lost her sense of reality. She had on her hat and coat and was carrying a handbag. She said she was going to see her mother (long since dead) and would they take her since they knew the road and she had forgotten it.

As my guests turned the corner toward North Hall, they heard loud, raucous shouts and laughter. Our Hungarian, Janos, was entertaining two children. To understand or even tolerate this confusion, one just has to know our Janos. He enjoys children so much. They adore him.

By this time Martha had also appeared on the scene. "Who are you visiting?" she shouted at Bob and Ruth. "Opal? Oh, Opal is a nice lady!" She ushered Bob and Ruth into my living room and tried to stay on with them. (I try to be tolerant with Martha. She has been deaf most of her life and has had very little company of her own.)

Before they could escape into my apartment, Amy, a most interesting ninety-six-year-old character, came in wearing one of her most flamboyant outfits. True to custom, she was guiding her wheelchair down the corridor and calling out "toot toot"! Oh, she has a fine mind for her age. But let's just say she is a bit eccentric, knows it, admits it, and enjoys it. I enjoy her, too. But Amy *is* a bit difficult to explain to newcomers.

As a grand finale to my guests' experiences, the worn-out, tired, old electric washer in the home's nearby laundry was turned on. It sounded much like an airplane tuning up! The three doors between the laundry and the corridor are usually closed. But not this day! (Since then we've gotten a new washer!)

To make the confusion even greater, Bob and Ruth were in so much of a hurry they really didn't have time to drink in the beauty of one of the most loved apartments in the Miami Valley—mine! How could I make them understand that when I close my apartment door I live in a world all my own? My closest companions are my color TV (Don't try to tell me you can't find any worthwhile TV programs!), an excellent stereo, two radios, a tape recorder, and a tape cassette player.

To these add some twenty color-slide programs of our travels for which I have taped our own narrations. I also have many other travel tapes I had fun making as my husband and I rambled along the byways, and twenty-five travel diaries I wrote about my memorable trips with my husband. They are typed and preserved in leather-bound notebooks, and make a nice addition to my bookcase.

Bob and Ruth also missed the perennial flower bed I have been struggling to grow. Two kinds of daisies, carnations, sweet williams, and the glorious sunflowers my grateful birds had planted for me were already in bloom. Soon there would be lilies, followed by perennial asters, sedum spectabile, and annual geraniums.

It was difficult to answer Ruth's question, "How on earth do you stand it here, Opal?" After all, they were here only about twenty minutes. After they described their entrance experiences, our brief minutes were filled with nostalgic references to our chance meetings while traveling. In such a short time, how could I explain that when you live in a nursing home you learn to understand older people in a deeper way?

I'm glad when people like me but I like doing things for them, too! We exchange favors and goodies to eat. We share! All year long, I write birthday, convalescent, and seasonal holiday cards for all the residents. I enjoy taking flowers to the sick and shut-ins. Going to rooms to pray with and for other residents who are ill helps me as much as it helps them.

How, in twenty minutes, could I tell Bob and Ruth about all the fine friends I have? About the wonderful gifts I receive in flowers, food, and stationery? How could I tell about the splendid care the nurses and their aides give me? I couldn't, not in twenty minutes.

Above all, I am never alone. God is always with me. I can talk to him in privacy whenever I want to. Often in the quiet hours we talk together. I believe in two-way prayer, which is a tremendous help to me.

There is peace in the solitude of my apartment. Here, in the shelter of God's love, is where I have my own personal, intimate devotions. Here I read my Bible, sometimes aloud, sometimes silently. Here is where I attempt to understand some resident who has shown cruelty and misunderstanding toward other kind souls. Here is where I try to understand why someone else deliberately tried to hurt me.

The privacy of my room offers a desirable place for private prayer with my most precious friends—my pastors, our administrator-chaplain, relatives—and even mere acquaintances. These sessions lift me up. From them I get the courage to forge ahead in spite of my physical handicaps.

That's how I stand it here! But my contentment did not come automatically. It took some special planning.

II

"If You Lif,
Old Is Vat You Git"

"So with old age is wisdom, so with length of
days, understanding. . . ."

Job 12:12

Because my grandfather spoke pure Pennsylvania
Dutch, a number of his quaint sayings became part
of our household. One was, "If you lif, old is vat you
git." Perhaps that's why, even in my youth, I knew
that planning for the future was not only wise, but
necessary.

When Laurel and I were first married, back in
1917, it took all my savings from two years of school-
teaching to buy our furniture. That was when I
decided to start another savings account for old age.
But not in the way most folks do it!

If I bought a dress or anything else—even
furniture—and for some reason did not keep it, the

refund money was deposited in my new savings account. I raised chickens and sold them the first summer we were married. The fifty dollars I cleared went into my savings.

I tutored high school students in the neighborhood who had failing grades, and put the money aside. When people gave me money for presents, I saved it. Occasionally Laurel would add money to my account, too. And there was a five-hundred-dollar inheritance from a distant aunt.

Through the years I held what they now call garage sales. The money I earned was often badly needed for other items, but if I could do without it, it landed in the growing retirement fund! These sales were especially outstanding during the Great Depression when there was little in the stores. That was when I got rid of wedding gifts I had sentimentally stored but never used!

My "trash" was someone else's treasure. I especially remember how much a prominent electrician reveled in the electrical equipment we had hung onto. And I can still see a young mother-to-be gratefully hugging an old-but-never-used washboard to her bosom. Nowhere had she been able to find one to use in their little apartment.

Each period of our married lives added its own contributions. Typical of post-World-War-II days were Laurel's beehives. As part of the war effort, he bought one beehive. Beehives have a habit of multiplying, and Laurel's assistant principal also brought him a colony he had found swarming in the nearby woods.

Laurel did not enjoy messing with the critters, though. So he gave them to his "honey"—me! How sweet of him! I detested working with bees, so I sold them, hives and all. They added dollars in the three columns to my fantastic savings account, which I continued to preserve for our retirement.

Most people dread old age. We tend to think of it as something that only happens to other people. Not us, we're not going to grow old. So we don't save for it, and we don't plan ahead. But the fact is, we do grow older. What are you going to do when that house and yard get too large for you to manage? Or if you've already moved to an apartment, what will you do with it if you become ill or injured? If you are happily married, have you contemplated and accepted the fact that one of you will one day be alone? Do you want to be independent, to avoid intruding into some loved one's happy family home?

Then no matter how young you are, it's not too soon to begin considering the alternatives. When a change becomes necessary, you may not be physically able to make inspection tours. Do you want someone else to solve the problem? If the solution is a retirement or nursing home, will you be happy if someone else selects it? How would you feel about being hauled off to a place you'd never seen? Adjustments are usually most difficult for those unfortunate souls forced to move to unfamiliar places without having any say in the matter.

Many people have not taken into consideration

that our life expectancy is much longer now. Statistics tell us that eleven percent of our population is over sixty-five years of age. Because childhood and adult diseases can now so often be treated, people are reaching their senior years in ever larger numbers.

In years past, several generations could live together in one house and support each other. Now, families and houses are smaller. A mother may be an invalid at eighty-seven, and her daughter or son can be anywhere from sixty-five to seventy years old and in failing health, too, or at least unable to care for an extra family member.

Our economic system and our increasing personal standards have almost forced all the adult members of an average family to become wage earners. A really good nursing home is therefore often the proverbial "godsend" when a person's ability to handle daily responsibilities wanes.

It was a real godsend to Laurel and me that we had looked at nursing homes some ten years before he died. We were prompted into this early study of nursing homes through the experiences of family and friends. Laurel's paralyzed sister had been in a splendid nursing home for many years. His former secretary, a dear friend to both of us, was in another home—the one where we later placed our application. And his assistant principal's widow was in a third one we thought was terrible.

It was realism, not negative thinking, that made us consider our future. We'd been married over forty years, and even if we'd had children, we would not have chosen to intrude on them. (We were both convinced that no house was built large enough for more than one family!) My health was fragile, and I had a heart condition, so we recognized the inevitability of nursing-home living. We began to study the possibilities.

What older people usually dread is having to leave their own homes. Staying with relatives does not remove that fear. Much depends on whether the person or couple is content, or even able, to stay alone. It sounds incredible to me, but I have met a few elderly parents who actually expected their adult children to give up their homes and move into the old family home with them!

If the older person has no physical or mental illness, daily visits from a family, church or club member may be the answer. The organization known as "Fish" does a lot for individuals who are in fair health, transporting them to the doctor, bringing them food and clothing, doing minor housekeeping chores, and making regular telephone checks.

Suppose a loved one could stay in his own home if he just had someone to cook good balanced meals for him. Then "Meals-on-Wheels," now provided in most areas by social agencies, is the answer.

Geography may have a lot to do with the solution you work out. Many farm communities in the middle west and in some eastern states have members of religious orders who still go into private homes to live and take care of the occupants. But this ideal solution is rapidly dying out. Factories in nearby towns pay better wages! Housekeepers, the old-fashioned practical nurses—yes, even neighbors and friends willing to live in—are becoming increasingly scarce.

You might be able to stay in your home and use a commercial day-care center. Usually a member of your family would take you to the day-care center in the morning and return you home at night. In most cases, however, "home" belongs to a relative.

Otherwise, the sale of your home is necessary, since most people need money to finance whatever alternative they decide on.

Ohio has government-subsidized housing developments. Low-income citizens live in one-story apartments strung out in long rows. It is something like living in one big house. The government requires residents to pay one-half of their income for rent. If you have already lived under similar conditions, you won't have many adjustment problems.

There are also boarding homes where families with a room or two to spare feed and shelter senior citizens. But these boardinghouses seldom become "real homes." Foster homes operate according to a similar plan as foster homes for children. More recently, organized residential-care and living-care centers have been developing. They are more like fancy nursing homes and offer skilled nursing care and therapy of all kinds—at a higher cost, of course.

What about going to live with a son or daughter, or some other relative? With most able-bodied members of the household away all day at work or school, this is not always an ideal solution, unless you can get a housekeeper or practical nurse to stay with you when no one else is home. In some cases, of course, you may be able to stay alone in the daytime, which certainly solves many problems.

My sister, Corrinne, and her husband kept our mother with them for several years before Mom finally chose to go to a nursing home. They were both teaching and were gone during the day, so they hired "sitters" for Mom. Just as they were going out in the morning, the phone would often ring.

"I have a sore throat today, so I can't stay with your mother."

"I'm sorry, but I have a family problem and I won't be able to stay with Mrs. Hutchins today."

Or some other reason.

Then Corrinne had to start down her list of some dozen substitute sitters until she reached one who could come. Sometimes no one was available.

There is no perfect answer. Laurel and I would much rather have stayed on at Glenside together but, knowing that the Lord might have other plans, we decided to sign up for a nursing home.

Actually, we applied to *two* good retirement-and-nursing homes in order to have priority if and when we needed one. We selected these two after visits to a number of homes in Ohio and Florida. Each year the homes checked with us, and my husband told them we were not ready to move.

"We are still able to take care of our house and each other," Laurel would say confidently. But he knew if anything unexpected came up we had a place to go.

27

We spent twelve wonderful years traveling and filling every moment of our retirement with new adventures. We did not sit at home in our rocking chairs. Instead, we kept looking at nursing homes from time to time and our minds were at ease.

Laurel had spent twenty-five years of his life as a high school principal. Now we were enjoying our retirement. How we enjoyed people in a new, liberated manner! No professional demands restricted us. We fished and boated. We beachcombed for sea shells, starfish, sea-horse skeletons, sand dollars, sponges, driftwood and coral.

I even took up acrylic painting as we traveled. Our bird-watching was magnified. Florida offered a bonanza in that field and was most kind to our cameras. While we relaxed and played and stretched our imaginations, our Dalmatian, Polka Dot, did everything we did.

Or should I say she copied everything we did on the beach? She brought us sea shells; she floated in the salt waters of the Gulf of Mexico and the Atlantic in an inner tube; she lay incumbent on her beach towel, stretched out like a person, not like a dog; she walked the beaches with both of us and raced her master on the sand in the spirit of frolic.

It was during that twelve-year honeymoon that Laurel and I grew so close to each other. ". . . And they shall be one flesh" (Gen. 2:24). We seemed more like one person—one extremely happy person—so in love that we would never be separated.

But we were separated—in a shockingly short

time. Spring was melting into summer, and Laurel was almost seventy-five. He'd noticed an annoying recurring discomfort in his gall-bladder region. Our doctor scheduled him for tests in the hospital.

The day before he left for the hospital, Laurel did a full day's hard work getting our acre-and-a-half of landscaping in perfect condition—and I do mean perfect. No one could groom a yard to perfection better than Laurel. He had the touch of a landscape artist, and Glenside "purred" at his touch.

For two weeks, diagnostic tests revealed nothing. Then severe pain set in, and the doctors decided that exploratory surgery was necessary. They found a pancreas full of cancer. It was a fast-growing malignancy.

As soon as my sister, Corrinne, and her husband, John, realized Laurel's condition, they went to the two nursing homes where we had our applications. They also looked at other homes, including the newly completed Valley Home. They felt that Valley outweighed all the others.

My heart had worsened rapidly that past year, and I also had thrombophlebitis in both legs. I had just spent seven months getting rid of deep-seated blood clots.

We knew that Laurel would not live through the winter, and Glenside was too large for me to manage at any season of the year. I would be alone now, and my health made it imperative for me to enter a care facility at my earliest convenience. John and Corrinne took me to see Valley firsthand. I knew it was the place for me. It fitted my needs better than either of the homes where we had applications, but I was grateful for the checking Laurel and I had done. Our research had helped to bring my needs into focus.

My first requirement was that my retirement home be near my family and friends. Valley Home is within a half-hour's drive of where I had lived almost all of my life, except during college and about four teaching years. I wanted a place with easy, ample parking for my guests. My preference was a small home, not an immense, cold institution.

My prayer was that it would be in the open country with grass and trees and open skies. A Christian home, rather than a purely commercial one, was more desirable. It must be capable of caring for me during an acute or terminal illness.

If I'd only had my school-teacher pension, then to be safe I would have taken a single room. But my "old-age account" had already grown to a $20,000 certificate of deposit, composed of sacrifice, work and FUN. My hard-working farm parents had also left an estate large enough that I knew I could easily manage to pay for an apartment. And Laurel had left me his life insurance and other savings.

The large apartment I saw at Valley was more than I had ever hoped for. All my family, including my in-laws, felt it was the best choice available for me since I had been used to large houses in the country all my life. So I placed a deposit on it.

I knew I could not move away from Glenside and let it stand empty, because I would constantly worry about vandalism. No room for sentiment now; I had to sell. Under less pressure my courage would have failed me, I am sure. Glenside was such a lovely home, so full of cherished memories. . . . The very day I knew that my Laurel could not live, I called a realtor.

"I want to list our Dutch Colonial home for sale," I explained. "It's forty-nine years old, and we built it in a hillside cornfield. There's an outdoor fireplace and a tennis court, a lily pond, brooks, and full-grown trees. The acre-and-a-half is fully land-scaped, and we have a Japanese bridge in one of the gardens. There's a three-car 'buggy shoppe.' " I offered to let the agent have it for sixty days only, telling him that it had to be sold by the last of September.

"If you'll give me a year, I can get $5000 more," he insisted.

"Two months," I repeated.

"Unheard of!" he countered.

"I also want to accompany you when you show Glenside to prospective buyers," I added.

"That's not often permitted." His voice sounded hesitant.

"Who knows Glenside's good points as well as I? And there's to be no dickering. The asking price and the selling price must be the same." The realtor acquiesced.

During Laurels' last days he knew his condition was terminal. It was a great comfort to him to know that my family had prevailed upon me to reserve an apartment at Valley Home. It was such a relief to him to know I would be taken care of. It made death easier for him. He could the more calmly say to me, "Sweetheart, I am going to have to leave you. But I'll wait for you in heaven."

The malignancy traveled with such speed that it soon ate through a large artery. Laurel started to hemorrhage, and within a few days he was mercifully gone. He had been in the hospital only four weeks.

Thursday morning, July 8, 1971, the hospital called to tell me that Laurel had just died. Then they called Miriam, my next door neighbor. When she found me a few minutes later, I was on my knees by the telephone desperately praying over and over, "Please, God, help me."

Yes, life has been good to me at Valley. The Lord answered that prayer.

III

It Helps to Be Prepared

"I have been young, and now I am old:
yet I have not seen the righteous forsaken."

Psalm 37:25

I buried Laurel on a Saturday. We made temporary arrangements for the sale of Glenside to a deserving young couple the following Tuesday. The material things of life were going well! How proud Laurel would have been of me!

Because we had faced reality through the fifty-four years of our married life together, I knew how to proceed even though I was absolutely frozen with grief and shock. (As I look back now, it seems as if I moved mechanically, like a robot.) We had long since bought our cemetery lot and monument and made written funeral arrangements, copies of which had been filed with our funeral director.

Of course our wills had been made years ago and revised several times. I was fortunate to have a qualified, honest attorney. I trusted him because he had handled our legal affairs before. But soon after I moved here his health failed.

Later I had my new attorney establish a trust fund to take care of my estate or handle my business in case I became incapacitated. We revised my will and made my funeral arrangements. Although it may be hard to handle these kinds of matters after a death in the family, they are essential business concerns that cannot be ignored.

Laurel and I had shared all business transactions, so I understood banking, check writing, and simple business in general. Every woman as well as every man needs to understand these basic business affairs.

More often it is the woman who has depended upon her husband, brother, or son to look after them for her. We have widows at Valley who don't know how to handle a checking account, much less invest and manage their moneys. They don't know how to deal with Medicare and other types of insurance.

Those were some of my responsibilities at Glenside, and I was grateful for the experience when I found myself alone. I had always helped with income tax and the monthly statements for our joint bank account. I was not entirely unprepared for the long road ahead.

I still had a twenty-eight-foot deluxe travel trailer, a station wagon, the furniture from the equivalent of a ten-room house, clothing, and household accessories to sell or give away. Meanwhile, the sale of my home furnishings had to be coordinated with the upcoming needs of my new home. I had to be careful not to sell something I would enjoy there. I worked steadily from mid-July to get ready to move on September 23.

First, I set up an "office" on our double bed: note pads, telephone directory, newspapers, and all the store catalogs I could get my hands on. From these catalogs I gleaned current prices as I lay on my "office bed." For articles classed as "used" furniture (rather than antiques), I charged about half price.

I nearly wore out the telephone checking current prices of silver and Spode, old books, and Currier and Ives prints, which were sold at full current value. After checking on prices, I informed my advisers that I had those items to sell and gave them my telephone number and directions for reaching me by car.

Then I asked Sally Gulasa, a fine high school girl who had helped us for the previous two years, to come every day that she could to "be feet for me." She carried all the small things for sale to the garage after I had put price tags on them. She arranged them on picnic and card tables and hung the clothing my family could not use on lines stretched in the buggy shoppe. Valuables like sterling, china, glassware, lamps, linens, and accessories were exhibited in the house and likewise price-tagged.

I had a dear friend, the proprietor of a reputable antique shop, who helped me, too. I had no auction.

I CHOSE TO LIVE IN A NURSING HOME

I didn't have the usual advertised garage sale. My publicity was by telephone and my many friends' word of mouth. I did run the risk of advertising my sterling flatware and Spode dinnerware in the newspaper.

There were times when I could not be on my feet at all to greet my would-be buyers. At those times I answered my callers through the intercom that went from my bed to our front door and told them what to do. They wrote down what they had chosen (on note pads I provided at the buggy shoppe), added up the cost, and paid me. To this day there are only a few small things for which I cannot account.

But toward the end I wore out heartwise, physically and spiritually, and I couldn't make it to the buggy shoppe any longer. In despair I called my only niece's husband and asked him to bring a truck to haul off to an auction whatever was left.

I still had to make insurance adjustments and changes in name and address for magazines, charge accounts, relatives, friends, business concerns, and bank accounts. Then I had to invest the money from the sale of the house, car, trailer, and partial furnishings. With all that accomplished, I thought now I must surely be finished with the ordeals of having to make decision after decision. But I was wrong!

My health demanded air-conditioning in my new apartment. There was already a built-in sleeve for it, but I had to find the make of one that would fit. To drain more of my energy, there was the smaller matter of choosing from the great array of telephones. A Princess telephone, which I could easily maneuver from my bedside table, was the answer. By then I was so fatigued that even choosing the color of the telephone was a chore.

But I was ready to move!

After three exasperating months of hurting, working, planning, and waiting, I was so relieved to have a reprieve that I rode away from Glenside without looking back, without shedding a tear. I could not yet believe it, but I was actually looking forward to my new apartment!

No, I would not try to deceive anyone into thinking I was brave. Oh, far from it! I hurt just as any one else would after having given up a deeply loved husband, a satisfying way of life, a treasured home. But I was so grateful to have Valley Home waiting for me, a home I would not have had if Laurel and I had not planned and prepared for it together.

Those last days of waiting at home by yourself are often the most traumatic period of all. It was three lonely months from the time Laurel died until I settled at Valley.

People came to visit, they telephoned, they sent flowers and notes of condolence, all of which helped to soothe my pain. But they did little to alleviate my burden.

Living in the country as I did, there were no relatives near enough to slip in often to look after me. Even had I been well enough to cook for myself, I would not have had the time. It was during this period that next-door neighbors came in to take care of me. Miriam and Andy Hanson carried trays of hot, luscious food to me every day from the first week of July until the last week in September. Due to our fenced-in country acreage, each trip to and from meant up and down three steep grades—a distance of probably an eighth of a mile. Carrying the trays was a feat. Indeed I appreciated and enjoyed the food on those trays—and the beauty of a flower bud in a vase or a thoughtfully included snack to hide in the refrigerator. But above all it was the presence of dear, true friends that relieved the monotony of loneliness and was miraculous healing for the great adjustment I had to make—being alone in a big house with numbers of almost unsurmountable tasks to perform.

On the other side of Glenside lived the Hammonds—my Dr. Hammond and his nurse-wife, Marian. It would be natural for my readers to think of them only in relation to my health. But all the time I was at Glenside alone they waited on me hand and foot. Every day they took my mail to and from my rural mailbox and carried my garbage out the long winding lane.

One of the fun things I remember was watching the dignified, handsome Dr. Hammond in his fatigues sling my large garbage bag across his shoulders and trudge down the lane with it. Quite a change in appearance from the man clad in his dark suit, carrying his doctor's satchel! There was not much fun in my life at that time, so I relished this episode.

IV

"I Came Here to Live"

When I was planning my move to Valley, I called to ask the interim administrator's permission to hang my own oil paintings on the walls.

"Just what all are you planning to bring?" he replied seriously. "We find that so many little old ladies want to bring too many sentimental keepsakes and things."

"I am *not* a little old lady and I *do* plan to bring lots of things," I retorted jokingly. "I plan to *live* at Valley, not just *stay* here. As to my paintings in oil and chalk, I would not class them as just 'things.' Most of them were done in art classes at college. I also took private lessons from Stutsman, who was with the Chicago Art Institute. These paintings have won acclaim in exhibits, and I would be most unhappy if I couldn't hang them in my new apartment."

This administrator had left Valley before I moved in, and I was relieved when the new administrator told me, "This apartment is your home. Do anything you like in it." So there are loads of lovelies in it for me and others to enjoy.

It was Corrinne and John who helped me move my things. John measured all the larger pieces of furniture and cut paper patterns to their size. (He used a roll of three-foot-wide dress pattern paper.) By laying them on the floor, we were able to tell which pieces of furniture we could bring to Valley. I found this more satisfactory than drawing floor plans or cutting small paper patterns to move about on a paper floor pattern.

I'm grateful that John went to the trouble of doing this for me, because I often hear my friends at Valley saying, "If I had only known, I could have brought along my bedside table and . . . and. . . ."

Corrinne hung all my oil paintings in their heavy frames, helped arrange furniture, and meticulously lined all chest and desk drawers with bright yellow-coated paper.

When I arrived at Valley, a prominent Dayton surgeon's mother lived across the hall from me in one of our single rooms (twelve feet by twelve feet in size). I visited her often and can still vividly see her room. She had a single bed and a bedside table on which she kept her clock, radio, and telephone. An electrified chaise lounge, a desk secretary, a large console TV, a lounge chair, a straight chair, three lamps, and an occasional table were her other furniture.

Many large and small pictures graced the walls, including pictures of her family. Small accessories, including several potted plants and three lamps, were placed around the room. There was little more than walking space left between things, but the effect of the whole was pleasing and attractive.

How much more comfortable than one single bed, one chair, and one chest of drawers—par for the course—for what many persons expect to and do bring here. But no one has to limit himself to such an austere decor. At least there can be familiar pictures on the walls, a reading lamp (for cheer if not reading), and possibly a radio and TV set.

These residents' eyes light up when they tell the stories of the extras in their rooms. Sometimes they can only point, or stare, at these familiar objects. Yet it seems to me that they are getting strength from them. I do!

Because I had been so insistent about bringing my lovely keepsakes to Valley, I was careful to meet all of the requirements of my new home. I wanted to be a good citizen and to make a good impression on our new administrator.

Then BOOM! The first week he arrived I overloaded an electic outlet and, of course, blew a fuse.

I felt like a naughty child but called the administrator immediately. He was kind and understanding, even though I had burned a wee hole in my carpet. He didn't scold one bit!

"Don't worry; no harm has been done." Then he checked all the outlets and wiring for me.

In appreciation I tried harder than ever to be a

model resident. Unfortunately, the electric fuse episode was not to be my last faux pas. I am persnickety about the carpet in my room. The nurse's aides had been carrying overly full glasses of cranberry juice from the door to my bed. They polka-dotted my gold-color carpet every inch of the way! It was at my request that the aides from then on were asked to carry snacks to the rooms on trays.

After all my ruckus raising, I did it! I spilled my *entire* glass of cranberry juice. I never realized how far a small glass of colorful, deep red fruit juice can travel! It did an amazing dye job on spread, sheets, pajamas—*and* carpet! The cheerful attitude of the aide who helped me clean up the mess was comforting.

I hadn't been at Valley very long before I realized that a comfortable adjustment to nursing-home living depended upon more than having understanding aides and keeping familiar objects in the room. Observing others, I became aware that those ten years of studying retirement and nursing homes with Laurel had paid off in other ways, too.

Some uninformed, unprepared people coming into a home for the first time get very upset—even to the point of confusion. I noticed that those who have been coerced by their families into coming here are much more difficult to get along with. Some even have ornery dispositions.

One woman said to me, "I ought to hate my son for bringing me here."

As we talked, Rachel admitted that her daughter-in-law could not possibly assume the extra responsibility of caring for her. She finally admitted it was the only thing her son had left to do. She even confessed that she liked Valley—although she had repeatedly said she hated it! The fact remained that Rachel was disturbed because she had not been consulted and shown the place ahead of time.

I have also witnessed some real trauma when senior citizens are denied the privileges they enjoyed in their own homes. But these dear people are not used to any kind of regimentation and had no idea they would run into it. I was grateful I'd become acquainted with the rules before moving to Valley.

There are state and federal laws for nursing homes, which, although good, and best for everybody's welfare, are upsetting. For example, medicine cannot be kept in individuals' rooms but must be kept in a locked area in the nurses' station and dispensed by the nurses, not the nurse's aides. Few people old enough or ill enough to be in a nursing home are capable of handling their own drugs.

One woman refused to stay in one of the best nursing homes in Ohio when she learned she could not keep her medicine in her own room. She forfeited her down payment and lost furniture-moving money as well as money paid for new furniture she could not use at her own home. In the end she had to settle for less satisfactory arrangements. And she still wasn't able to keep medicine in her room!

Some other common rules are elimination of all safety hazards such as electrical cords placed where they might cause falls, overloaded outlets, faulty wiring of lamps and appliances, open uncontrolled space heaters, and extension cords. (No cooking appliances are permitted in residents' rooms at Valley.)

Some time ago a sharp state inspector was in my room looking for safety hazards. I was flattered as he stood near my sea shell collection and admired it over—and over—and over—well, long enough to write his report that I had an electric space heater in my apartment. (It was near the sea shells, of course.) He said nothing to me about the heater, which at the time I didn't even know was a forbidden appliance. As he was leaving, he continued his comments on what a lovely apartment I had. And I basked in the many compliments as usual.

Our administrator was the first to see the written report. He has a sense of humor, too. Our tactful inspector had also caught a space heater in the nurses' station!

Some new residents bring a lot of pretty scatter rugs. When they learn they cannot keep the rugs, they go into a mental spin. Better that kind of spin than a fall and broken bones resulting from tripping over a treasured but dangerous scatter rug.

One of our residents had to give up a beautiful but flammable wastebasket for a metal container, which is more fire resistant. The resident loved that basket. "It was a gift from my great-granddaughter," he wept. "She is just seven years old. Prettiest blue eyes you ever did see. Why can't I keep it?" Tearfully he sobbed this out to the administrator, who feared the old gentleman might sneak a cigar occasionally and drop the burning butt into the basket.

None of these things surprised me, because the literature from all the nursing homes we studied had prepared me for them. My common sense confirmed the need to honor the rules.

Yet there were some adjustments I did have to make. Hardest of all, of course, was learning to live without my husband in new surroundings and with strange people. Fortunately, I meet people and make friends easily. That helps. Even so, like most people, I've never been used to people from all walks of life stepping directly and often unannounced into my bedroom.

There are inspectors, painters, dry cleaners, TV repairmen, nurses, aides, lab technicians—even visitors! But now I've learned to welcome those interruptions; I need them.

I also needed some help with transportation. While some homes make better arrangements than others, transportation for one who is semiambulant is no doubt a major adjustment problem at any nursing home.

Remembering that we usually become more helpless as the years add up, one thing I did to prepare myself was to patronize local services. For instance, I changed to a local dentist, a local optician and local attorney. The first two provide services in their offices and I have to go there in person. When I need the services of my attorney, though, he stops at my apartment on his way past Valley.

Some residents find shopping a real problem. I

was always so busy with family, church, school, and clubs that I learned to shop by telephone and mail. That was a long, long time ago. Now it has become a popular custom with many smart shoppers.

Since I have been at Valley, I do most of my shopping by telephone and thus save time, energy, and money for something more important and enjoyable. Besides the two old Chicago standbys, there are now many new reputable catalog stores that offer excellent services. A catalog, a telephone, a regular charge account (one that must be paid at the end of each month), mail delivery, and the package is mine. Ordering can be done by mail, too.

When local stores advertise in the newspaper, they are just as near as the telephone. They deliver the packages to customers' doors. If the merchandise proves undesirable, most local stores will pick it up for a reasonable charge. Valley also has church volunteers who occasionally shop for residents.

The families or attorneys of most Valley residents manage their business affairs for them. I still take care of my own by telephone or mail. But my trust company is ready to take over when I no longer can. My teacher's pension is sent directly to my bank checking account after the State Teachers Retirement System of Ohio has deducted my Medicare fee. I have not gone to a bank in person since I have been at Valley; even my certificates of deposit are handled by telephone and mail.

Another adjustment Christians have to make when moving to a nursing home is in the area of religion. One of the reasons I had chosen Valley in

46

the first place was that it was a church-related home. Seventeen churches of the same evangelical Protestant denomination support Valley Home.

I've had fairly close relationships with the parent churches since I was a teenager, almost seventy years ago. My father-in-law was a minister in one of them. After Laurel and I were married, we attended one of their colleges together, though we became Presbyterians early in our marriage.

I thought I would fit in perfectly. After all, I shared their basic belief in God and heaven. I had been aware of their viewpoint over a long period of time. Even so, having been a Presbyterian for over forty-five years, I was most surprised to encounter a bit of uncomfortable difference at first.

Some of the residents who were members of the sponsoring churches were most positive I would not go to heaven if I did not join their church. Of course, I could not go along with that! I do not even feel that way about my own church!

There were other church-oriented adjustments concerning dress, cosmetics, and recreation to which I paid little or no attention, although I was very much aware of them. For example, to the best of my knowledge, I was the very first woman resident to come through the front doors in a pantsuit, and that did not meet complete approval.

In fact, one of the "saints," whom the nursing staff could not persuade to wear panties and stockings when she left her room, kept quoting Deuteronomy 22:5 to me: "The woman shall not wear that which pertaineth unto a man . . . for all that do so are abomination unto the Lord thy God." Just a couple of years later pantsuit uniforms for women staff members were approved by the board of trustees and some of the trustees' and ministers' wives were coming to Valley in pantsuits!

Even though my new home is sponsored by a church whose customs varied a bit from those of my denomination, we all believed in the same God, the same Bible, the Holy Trinity, and baptism. In fact, as far as I was concerned, we agreed on all the important beliefs. I suspect that my "religious" adjustment to Valley was easier than the adjustment some of the people had to make for me!

One of the reasons some people are unhappy in nursing homes is that they have nothing to do and nothing to think about. They sit in uncomfortable chairs begging God to take them. They talk only about their troubles and make others miserable.

Would that they had become involved in building a reservoir of spirituality and deep religious character to lean upon—something within themselves to take wherever they go.

When I walk or buzz down our long hallway in my motorized wheelchair, I often see some of the older people quietly reading their Bibles or noisily listening to the religious programs on TV or radio; I can actually feel the comfort they are receiving. And this keeps them content. We can all find help in adjusting by looking upward.

One other big factor in adjustment concerns the failure to develop special activities and hobbies in earlier life. Moreover, it is not unusual to find residents refusing to start a new activity once they have entered a care facility. Often these are the very persons who failed to furnish soul, mind, and spirit with dimension and sparkle in earlier years. Not having valued living beyond a mere existence in younger years, they fail to recognize that during retirement, and even after failing health, all of us are given a splendid time to expand activities and to make old interests more meaningful than ever.

I have found that the best antidote to difficult adjustments is just to consider them a challenge. Because I can do all things through Christ who strengthens me, I am able to handle these adjustments. After all, I didn't come here to wait for death. I didn't come here for an extended "stay." I came here to live!

V

Where We Live

The traffic-busy highway in front of our acreage here at Valley was once known as Buttermilk Falls Road. Members of the Wenger family who used to farm this land tell me that the Buttermilk Falls are still bubbling about three hundred yards west of the present highway. They are on the Buttermilk Falls Creek, which forms our north boundary. Our one-story building of Early American architecture sits well back toward the center of twenty-two grassy acres.

Our tall flagpole proudly holds the flag of the United States. It stands majestically near the building where we can all see it. I love to watch from my windows when a determined breeze unfurls it. When the wind is lazy, Old Glory trails gracefully down along the flagpole.

The horseshoe-shaped entrance lanes and parking areas are ample. Even when there is traffic, they are wide enough to accommodate residents out for a walk. Wheelchair patients also appreciate our blacktopped surfaces.

In addition to the main marquee entrance, there are exits and entrances at both ends of the long hallways, and doors opening onto the vegetable and flower gardens and roofed patio. These six exits and entrances surely make life more pleasant and comfortable for us. They help us enjoy life outside the building. If we want a short walk, there is a doorway close by. A long walk? That is possible, too. If we begin to tire too much, no matter which door offers refuge, there is always a chair waiting for us just inside.

On these walks there are many delightful things to see: the fountain garden, the foundation plantings of taxus evergreens, borders of brilliant flowers back of the building, many spring flowering trees—plum and cherry and crab apple.

Far to the rear is a baseball field used by the young people from the churches that built Valley Home. Near the diamond is a twenty-six-by-forty-three-foot roofed picnic shelter. Eventually, a few wheelchairs may be able to reach it by way of a surfaced path, yet to be built. This picnic shelter was funded by memorial gifts. Joe, our administrator, says he knows of no other home with such a feature.

Eight cottages with the same chaste Early American architecture as the main building provide independent living facilities and another level of care at our retirement village. They are most popular and are proving our best source of income.

The homey entrance foyer is not plush, but it is in practical good taste, as is all our building. Visitors tell me they feel at home immediately.

Unless they are meeting with guests or waiting for transportation, Valley discourages residents from sitting in the entrance foyer. This request makes it most alluring!

Built to house a maximum of fifty residents, Valley Home has fourteen single rooms, seventeen doubles, and one apartment. Our home has three lounges, two of which are equipped with television. North Lounge is kept quiet so those with guests may have a larger secluded place in which to visit.

The most popular gathering place is our Fireplace Lounge located just back of the foyer. It is used mostly by wheelchair and walker patients who "watch" TV while they sleep. For safety's sake the logs in the fireplace are make-believe and the flames are artificial, but some of us actually feel warm just looking at them because we pretend they are real. There has been no run on the books in the built-in bookcase, which stretches halfway across the wall. Perhaps that's because we have such splendid bookmobile service from the Dayton-Montgomery County Library.

In the bookcase corner of the Fireplace Lounge there is a thirty-gallon fish aquarium, aestetically planned with growing plants and enlivened with tropical fish. It is good therapy just to gaze meditatively into its beauty and mystery. I am entranced when the incoming water makes the tropical plants wave and sway in correlated symmetry. And who can resist watching the graceful curves and flashing colors of the ever-active fish?

In another corner of the Fireplace Lounge is what we jokingly call "the bar." It was planned for residents who wish to toast bread, make a quick cup of coffee, or prepare for guests. Cupboards with dishes, hot plates, and electrical outlets are available in the bar.

I am so grateful they don't allow cooking in our rooms, since it could be dangerous. Neither would I enjoy the offensive floating odors of onions, cabbage, or burnt beans. Valley has the reputation of being as free from offensive odors as any nursing home could possibly be. Visitors have mentioned this to me many times.

As in all well-equipped nursing homes, there is an intercom system over which we can call the nurses and they can call us, individually. There is also an all-call system over which the nursing station may reach all residents' rooms at the same time for public announcements.

The public address system in the administrator's office only goes through the hallways. It is frequently used to broadcast seasonal music throughout the building. When we want to listen to the music, all we have to do is open our doors.

Anyone who wants to may have his own private telephone. That way calls don't have to come through an office switchboard.

We are well set up for communication, so we have

no problem communicating! We even have a fire bell system. It is so sensitive that the alarm bell goes off when a kitchen employee burns the toast! It is not a nuisance, however, since it can be turned off manually. The alarm goes off, too, whenever the fire sprinkler in any part of the building goes into action.

An approved sprinkler system has been installed throughout the building. Ours is a dry system, which means that there is no water in the ceiling sprinklers, only air.

To activate the sprinklers in the ceilings of my apartment, there would have to be enough heat to melt the wax material in one or more of my room's sprinklers. The air in the pipes would then be released so the water could enter and start to sprinkle. No other sprinklers in the building would be set into action unless the fire spread to the hall or other rooms. That is almost impossible because most fires can be put out by less than five sprinklers.

I like our one-story building. I dread the thought of multi-story nursing homes. Here I can crawl out of one of my windows in case of a fire!

In each of our rooms we enjoy the comfort of electric heat with individual thermostatic control. Instant heat. Instant turnoff. The building is centrally air-conditioned. Each resident's room has its own built-in sleeve where, if he wants it, the resident may install his own air conditioner.

The master communal TV aerial is provided with an outlet for individual TV hookups in each room as well as in the three lounges. We furnish our own TV set. Residents have no maintenance worries of any kind. We don't even have to replace our own light bulbs!

Each resident's room has its own private bath. (Some older nursing homes still have common bathrooms, however.) The floors and lower bathroom walls are ceramic tile—a sanitary as well as a safety asset.

It would not be a fully equipped nursing home without offices for the administrator and his secretary, a nursing station, a doctor's examination room, a kitchen and activity room, of course.

The small building and small enrollment contribute, I am convinced, to my sense of being part of one big, friendly family. It is small enough that I can be aware of the health of the other residents and pray for them individually.

Each noon before meals the administrator brings a devotional. He tells us who is ill and who is in the hospital, and informs us of their progress. As the birthdays of residents occur, he wishes them a happy birthday.

Once each month a nearby church bakes and decorates a birthday cake large enough for all the residents. The activity director plans a monthly birthday party for all of us in honor of those whose birthdays fall in that month.

The tables in our well-appointed dining room are round and accommodate four people on attractive (but very uncomfortable!) captain's chairs. I remedy this discomfort with my own extra cushion, as do many others. (I would like to pass on a bit of caution to any trustee who might have the burden of choosing chairs for a nursing home: SIT in one your-self for an hour before you buy!) Thanks to one faithful resident, our tables always have center-pieces: fresh flowers, artificial flowers, small plants or novelties made by local church and club groups.

The south wall of the dining room is a solid row of Early American windows. Through these windows in spring, summer and fall, we can see the flower-bordered concrete walkways that lead to the foun-tain. The symmetrical, well-tended garden is a glad-some sight. Today as I write, buxom pumpkins weighing up to fifty-two pounds add the warmth of lambent orange to the cool greens and dying browns. They forecast Halloween a comin'!

We are fortunate at Valley because we live where there are more trees than people. Probably the most restful of all sights from our dining room windows is the distant panorama of full-grown deciduous trees along South Brook, which give the home a genuinely rural atmosphere in all seasons. They ease tensions, heal hurts, smooth angers, and bring tranquility.

The dining room doubles as an assembly room, as is the case in many modern buildings. The front portion incorporates a piano, organ, and microphone-equipped lectern flanked by both the United States and Christian flags. A chaste walnut cross suspended on the drapery-covered wall be-hind the lectern, looks protectively down upon us, lest we forget.

VI

I'm in Love Again

Laurel and I were deeply in love with Glenside. I thought nothing could ever take its place. But I'm in love again—this time with my apartment! I can honestly say that it stands at the top of the list of those things that have most helped me to adjust to nursing-home life. Furnished cozily with things brought from Glenside, the apartment has become my home.

It's really the size of four good-sized rooms, but they have been combined into two large rooms. Almost everything in the rooms is from Glenside, from the Sollenberger family crest hanging on the outside of the door to the solid walnut schoolmaster's desk that sits across the room in front of a four-and-a-half-by-nine-and-a-half-foot picture window. Modern brass floor lamps at each end accent the desk's antiquity.

On the south wall of the living room are my two walnut pedimental corner cupboards. There are no suitable corners in the apartment for them, so my clever sister suggested that they stand together as one piece of furniture, mid-wall. They are comfortably filled with some of my collectors' items—mainly old glass and china.

Two large mid-Victorian, hand-carved rose-and-grape armchairs look most substantial. For anyone who wishes to be dignified, they are good to sit in, too! Then there is the little rose-carved occasional chair some guests choose. I did the needlepoint for its seat. Other visitors prefer one of the maple occasional chairs that rest at either end of my mother-in-law's large curly-maple and curly-walnut drop-leaf wedding table.

Many cunning little creatures live with me in my apartment. There are Swedish glass birds, a Staffordshire china bird from England (via Bermuda), and a ceramic bird from Japan. There are silken embroidered horses from old China and painted wooden horses from Sweden that stowed away in airplanes with my sister and her husband. I am especially in love with my sculptured bronze lambs and the tall, lanky, Egyptian-looking turquoise cats from old China.

I enjoy gazing at the carefully sculptured bronze owl that "flew" onto Laurel's desk on the twenty-fifth anniversary of his high school principalship. There's also a hand-carved wooden elephant from Thailand; a knotty little frog from Japan; a dark teakwood bird from near Mount Kilimanjaro, in Tanzania; and a sly little applewood rabbit from the Smoky Mountains.

Together with my twenty-four-inch console color TV, my traditional sofa serves as a room divider. It is soft, friendly, and inviting. Behind the sofa on the den side is a large sturdy coffee table I made from our first piano bench.

The natural light on the den side of my apartment is splendid. It has the same large windows as the living room. My hospital bed has a quaint Shaker Patch coverlet of brown and natural, and its head is rolled up so it resembles a chaise lounge.

My den houses some of my favorite books on opera, art, interior decoration, Early American furniture, nature, and travel. Most of the books are in the bookcase that also holds an interesting, old, tall, New Haven mantel clock. I store my overflow of purposefully good books in an old, copper washboiler. I'll never forget the day I bought it from old Bert, a local antique dealer. The washboiler was completely covered with a black smoke deposit; not a hint of copper shone through. One of my bobby pins sneaked out and "diagnosed" the metal as copper. Much to Laurel's consternation, I slipped Bert a dollar bill and the copper *objet d'art* appeared in our car. It took me about a year to get it cleaned and polished. Each time I went to the basement to put clothes in the washer or dryer I took a little whack at it. Was my husband proud of the resulting valuable antique—all for one dollar!

I have always found my color scheme—aqua and

rose—so satisfying that I have carried it out in my bathroom, too. I've hung paintings of our rose-colored tulips and the aqua water lilies that grew at Glenside. A map of the United States, which I hand-painted for our first Trotwood travel trailer, hangs in the shower room. Its aqua frame carries out my color scheme and gives life to a large portion of the top back shower wall. I've also added an aqua-and-rose fruit plate that belonged to my great-grandmother. I feel pleased to have my bathroom decorated just as nicely as the rest of my apartment.

My best loves are my four roomy closets. All of them have furniture stored in them. Clothing hangs on either side under the shelves or on top of the low furniture. The first closet in my bedroom contains a dressing table made from an old pine writing desk, a triple folding mirror, and an old Shaker chair Laurel's father made.

The chair and table really convert the closet into a little dressing room. The second closet holds a chest of drawers topped with several large loaded suit-cases. I can almost hear the shelves groaning under their heavy burdens!

In one entrance hallway closet I have a small re-frigerator on top of a four-drawer chest. The shelves of the fourth closet are laden with movie film, color-slide pictures, with their corresponding tape recordings, and other photographic equipment. I recorded the tapes one spring when Laurel drove me out to the quiet Florida countryside few tourists ever see.

The soft, rich, neutral gold of my wall-to-wall

carpet helps absorb all the colors of my lovelies. I've combined primitive, Early American, Victorian, modified mid-Victorian and just-plain-modern furnishings. Nothing is as boring or uninteresting as a room all furnished in one period.

If you are about to move into a nursing home, I'd suggest you make your room attractive and comfortable. Don't sell your furniture and accessories before you are absolutely sure you can't use them. A few of the things I have heard our residents say they wish they had saved include: flower vases, pictures, lamps, chairs, cushions, footstools, small tools, bed linens, towels, jewelry boxes, storage chests, a small desk.

There is an unusually high correlation between a nursing-home resident's ability to adjust to his new life and the way his room is furnished. In fact, I know of only three people who have furnished their rooms with mementos from their previous home who are unhappy with being in a nursing home.

Size is not important. Two of the happiest people have attractively decorated and furnished two of the smallest rooms in the home. But there are also several bare, uninteresting, underfurnished rooms with no pictures on their walls and no knickknacks—not even a reading lamp! Ninety-some percent of the people in those rooms are restless, unhappy, cantankerous, and generally miserable.

Laurel and I had drawn our own plans for Glenside. We did most of the supervision during its construction. As the years passed we added to the home touches that made it distinctively our own. Glenside was an extension of us. Perhaps that's why it's almost a serendipity that I could so easily transfer my love to this apartment and adjust as well and quickly as I did.

Yes, I'm in love again!

VII

"Not by Bread Alone"

Mmm—I always dreamed how elegant it would be to have the luxury of breakfast in bed. But how different it is when health necessitates the service! For some reason my pulse races so fast in the early morning that my doctor made arrangements for me to stay in bed for breakfasts. My typical low-fat breakfast menu includes orange juice, toast and jelly, hot cereal, one banana, dry skim milk, whites of two poached eggs, and a hot drink.

The monotony is occasionally relieved by French toast or pancakes with syrup, and, once in a while, by scrambled eggs. On Sunday we get a scrumptious piece of coffee cake, a sweet roll, or a doughnut. Our genial, cooperative ex-marine chef sends me a surprise goody now and then. This morning it was a bacon-stuffed omelet. Yummie!

For those who go to the dining room, breakfast at

Valley is unique. Residents may go to the dining room any time between eight and nine o'clock. They concoct their own breakfast menu from all Valley offers, which gives them a wide choice. The nurse brings their medicines to the tables, as she does for all meals.

As should be, we have our heaviest meal at noon. The same menus are served to all residents, except where special diets must be followed. Today I had ham, whole wheat bread, grape jelly, sweet potatoes, green beans, cake and a canned pear.

We fill out individual menus for supper several days in advance. We choose between the "either-ors," and if we are not on a strict diet or fussy about what we eat, these supper menus offer a full meal. Here is an exact copy of a supper menu:

Celery soup ___ or Vegetable beef soup ___
Crackers ___ bread ___ jelly ___
Peanut butter and jelly sandwich ___
   or Ham sandwich ___
Cottage cheese ___ or three-color jello cubes ___
Ice cream ___ or glorified rice ___
Cold cereal ___
Milk ___ hot water ___
Coffee ___ Sanka ___ hot tea ___
Iced tea ___ hot chocolate ___

Daily snacks come mid-morning, mid-afternoon and at bedtime. Fruit juices, crackers, cookies, ice cream, hot chocolate, milk, or whatever choices our doctor permits are served in our rooms. No one need go to bed hungry here at Valley. I am a weight watcher. That is why I ask for a snack at bedtime only.

Adjusting to food is a big problem at any nursing home. When there are dozens of residents, the kitchen cannot cater to each individual's likes and dislikes. Because Laurel and I had been visiting homes and eating in their dining rooms, I was better prepared to adjust when I moved into Valley.

When I first came here the thing that rankled me most was the way they served the food. For example, sloppy spinach or broccoli or kale liquid ran across the plate to socialize with the mashed potatoes and chicken. But hear ye, hear ye, one of my tablemates, a retired nurse, used to send the waitress back to the kitchen for more "broth" on her vegetables. She was right; the minerals and vitamins were in that liquid.

But I prefer the vegetables served in side dishes that retain these nutritious liquids. Again, however, there is a reason why Valley does not offer this nicety. As are most homes, they are understaffed in the kitchen, and slapping the "greens" on the dinner plate saves time and dishwashing!

Not every resident responds to dining room and food problems in the same way. A lot depends upon what the residents have been used to. If they pampered themselves with huge steaks at home, then glorified hamburger just isn't going to be their cup of tea. If they doted on hand-embroidered linens, coordinated centerpieces and dinner music supplied by classical stereo recordings, they will note a big difference in the atmosphere of a nursing home's group dining room.

Then there is the problem of methods of cooking food. For instance, you may like your vegetables in a cream sauce, but the home serves them plain in order to honor certain individuals' diets. You may not like plain-cooked vegetables, but they are better for an older person's health.

Many are accustomed to a lot of salt. This presents an adjustment necessitated by the fact that many doctors order salt-free diets. We learn to add salt at the table; and if we are determined to do so, we can learn to like salt substitutes. Nursing-home residents find a happy bonus in a low-salt or salt-free diet because it helps them to reduce—and who isn't trying to reduce in this age of physical fitness? Moreover, many of the best restaurants now serve salt-free foods, so you don't have to feel penalized by nursing-home requirements.

The transfer from independent living to residency in an institution creates its own special set of food adjustments. On the first crisp fall day who doesn't develop a yen for pumpkin pie, or sauerkraut and sausage, or even hot chocolate? In your own kitchen you could promptly proceed to satisfy that desire.

However, once you are a resident in a home, you can't satisfy your every whim. We are hungry for certain food at different times. We don't get it quite when we might want it. Too, some days the cooks just miss the boat! That's the day I secretly count on my fingers how much I'm paying for that unappetizing meal.

But wait a minute. When I cooked at home, not everything always turned out just as I wished either. And I've gone to a restaurant where I raved about the food, but when I returned at a later time, I found the food most disappointing. I have relatives and friends whose cooking I don't like, but I keep on accepting their invitations even though their coffee is bitter.

I have to laugh at some of the oft-reiterated remarks the older men make about the food.

"I never saw potatoes fixed like that, don't even look like potatoes."

"In all the years I lived with Esther she never cooked anything like this."

Most people can learn to like certain foods if they set their minds to it. Some are just too stubborn to try. They remind me of children who never tasted certain foods because they knew they didn't like them. I find this silly attitude expressed more often by men than by women. (Call me a female chauvinist if you will!)

So often when people live alone, they don't eat properly. A home takes care of that problem to a great extent. The dietician at a home will see to it that residents eat what the doctor specifies where special diets are indicated. Most people cheat on their diets when they live at home and thus miss an opportunity to improve their health. Many times a new home resident's health improves. Some of our skinny people here actually gain weight. Of course, some of the already fat ones do, too!

Food should be kept covered, anywhere. By law,

it must be tightly covered in your room at a home to prevent ants and other insects as well as dust from getting to it. Perishable foods are taboo unless refrigerated. Some new patients rebel and break these laws. Then they feel they are abused when corrected.

Once a brand-new, young nurse on her first stint of active service at Valley saw me carrying a slice of bread and packet of jelly from the dining room table to my apartment. We have a rule that prohibits residents taking food to their rooms unless they have their own refrigerators. Terry had not been here long enough to learn that I am required to eat lighter meals at the table and supplement the diet between meals, nor did she realize I had a refrigerator in my apartment.

She chased down the corridor after me, calling excitedly, "Oh, Opal, you are taking food to your room." Her wobbly pursuit was all the funnier since she was very much pregnant, and the prospective baby was reaching me before she was!

There is no denying the day-in and day-out monotony of eating institutional food, usually with little choice of menu. That's why most ambulant patients delight in being taken out to a restaurant to eat. One of the ladies who used to work at Valley as a volunteer recognizes this. Eleanor Whitesell has become more than a volunteer to me; I cherish her friendship.

She has taken me out frequently to restaurants to eat, but I enjoy lunch at her family home better. It is like helpful medicine to sit by her windows and look out over the valley and lake.

The late Janet Day, one of Valley's former outstanding head nurses, took me to her home at least three times for lunch. People have no idea what it means to be a guest in a real-for-sure home when you are living in an institution. Her home was comfortable, relaxed, friendly, usable. I wasn't afraid to lie down when heart fatigue began.

The first thing I noticed when we drove up to her home was the bird feeder, at which two cardinals were feasting. Then many flowers nodded their welcome to me. Beyond the flowered backyard was a vegetable truck patch—not just a garden! What fun it was one sunny afternoon to help Janet pull their homegrown elderberries from the stems as I lounged on a chaise on the comfortable back porch.

Sometimes it's not possible to take a resident out to a restaurant or home to dinner, but my family and friends have discovered the next best thing! Corrinne brings food gifts with her when she comes to visit. They are always unusual.

Sometimes it's washed lettuce from her garden, wrapped in zippered cellophane bags. She adds my favorite salad dressings as a bonus. Other times she prepares cantaloupe, watermelon or honeydew melon in cellophane-wrapped meal-sized slices. And chocolate pudding in throwaway containers tantalizes me!

A young friend, Gail Lindsay, who had been a beautician at Valley's Beauty Shop, called me each time she came over to ask if she could stop at any of the stores for me. She always brought me little bits to eat—a piece of pie or cake, an apple or a bunch of grapes. Twice she brought me a complete hot lamb dinner that she had prepared and packed so well they lost none of their warmth. I missed her for a few weeks and was stunned when I heard she had died of cancer. She had lived so much in her short life!

One time my younger brother, Myron, and his wife, Jo, had driven miles to pick domestic black raspberries. That evening they dropped in to surprise me with them—and some shortcake! I couldn't help eyeing the plump, luscious fruit from time to time during their visit. After Jo and Myron left, I plunged into the juicy berries and shortcake with unmoderated delight.

My friends and family are careful to check with the head nurse before they bring me any kind of food gift. That way there is no danger of going outside my restricted diet. They avoid candy, nuts, and rich foods. They are not good for older persons and are denied on most diets.

If we don't eat the food before they leave, my friends make sure there is a way to cover it tightly. They try to use disposable containers. If the food is perishable, the nurse's aides at Valley will put it in the central refrigerator at the nurses' station if a resident does not have his own.

It isn't just the difference between institutional food and "outside" food that makes these treats so special. It's the extra touch of love that goes with them. Somehow these extras, the manna of God's love and concern, renew and uplift me.

One sunny morning Rey, a former nurse at Valley, called me to tell me she was going down to a fruit stand in the country for strawberries. Would I like to go along? Would I! She thoughtfully planned our excursion along the most come-hither side roads and pointed out things of interest to me. She also drove me past places that live in my memory: my birthplace, my second home, my home of forty-nine years that I left to come to Valley. . . .

It was the first time in years I had had the opportunity to browse among fruit and vegetable stands. It would be most difficult for anyone else to understand the thrill of just buying a tomato!

It took so little, but it did so much to make me happy!

VIII

Rx for Boredom

If I have one complaint to voice, it is that there are
only twenty-four hours in a day! No one can ever
say that I've been bored. There are new adventures
and favorite pastimes, new experiences, and comfortable routines to greet me every single day.

Every noon meal begins with an announcement
from the podium of the day of the week, the month,
the date, and the year. If the day is a holiday, the
announcer adds an appropriate comment. These
before-lunch announcements are helpful in keeping
residents oriented to time. Most of their calendars
are not filled with enough appointments to keep
them aware of the date. But just this morning the
host on one of the three major TV networks used the
wrong date, and he does not live in a nursing home,
either!

I CHOSE TO LIVE IN A NURSING HOME

My breakfast tray arrives between seven thirty and eight while I am still in bed. Usually I have been up just long enough to brush my teeth, wash my face and hands, and possibly do a bit of grooming. Other times I may greet the aide's pleasant, "Good morning, Opal!" with curlers in my hair. I set no alarm clock.

The aide who carries in my tray brings my newspaper (which has already been put on the handrailing outside my door). She also takes any outgoing mail to the mailbox in the foyer, in order to catch the morning mail.

After breakfast, I take my daily sponge bath, unless this is one of the three mornings reserved for real brush-scrubby showers. Those residents who cannot shower or take tub baths by themselves are given this care by the aides twice a week. Both the daily bather and the one who thinks Saturday night is the only time for baths must become accustomed to this change in procedure.

An aide makes my bed each day, and every Wednesday she changes the linens, which I am requested to furnish. On Tuesday evening an aide does my flat laundry (bedding and towels), plus my pajamas and robes. I do all my own hand laundry, including lingerie, hosiery, good dresses, and good sweaters. The aides do all this for those who are unable to do their own—as well as for some who could do their own! In many cases, a family member takes the laundry home.

By Friday my apartment needs a thorough cleaning, so the regular housekeeper vacuums the carpet, dusts, and scrubs the bathroom. Window washing is an occasional treat. The housekeeper empties the waste cans daily. We pay no extra charge for these cleaning services. It is my job to keep my closets, desks, corner cupboards, and tabletops neat.

I also have appointments for a shampoo and set at Valley's beauty shop on Fridays. This service is available to residents at a modest additional charge. That's where I learn what's going on! One lady, who is an avid reader and "hooked" on mystery stories, always brings her own books to read. Another is diligently knitting a well-turned sweater of royal purple yarn. Some sleep. Oh, how they sleep! A few take advantage of the magazines and eagerly leaf through the assorted gift catalogs in the shop.

Those who have few guests welcome the sociability of Valley's beauty shop. Like all beauty shops, ours is a good place for visiting. Bea, a lonely lady who loves to talk, regularly stops at the shop to kibitz several times during the days the beautician is on duty.

When she is under the dryer, she reads religious books and periodicals. Reminiscing about her past, she tells winsome stories about the children in the families for whom she worked as a housekeeper. She knows the names of all the staff and residents and facts about their families. Her knowledge is helpful to other residents who do not remember names. One day I spoke of something amusing one of my grandnephews had done. I was surprised to hear her question, "That's Linda's little boy, Harris, isn't it?" It gives me a warm feeling to know that another resident cares that much.

We have colossal expectations of the hairdresser's art. I would like my hair to look like a TV star's. Impossible! A very old lady in the home wants her hair cut just like mine with a close shingle and a severe point at the nape of the neck. But the poor dear does not have enough hair to cut! Her pink scalp makes much more color than her white hair. Imagine a couple of dozen elderly ladies all wanting a beauty operator to do their hair exactly as it was done years ago "back home"!

It is amazing to watch the dexterity and patience with which the hairdressers handle wheelchair patients and those on walkers. A derrick has to be used to transfer some of the patients from wheelchair to shampoo chair. Some are lifted with the help of one or two nurse's aides.

Most do not mind. Just getting transferred from their room to the shop is a happy change. Since some residents seldom leave their rooms, just seeing a new face is a special delight. To have someone, anyone, waiting on and serving them is comforting.

However the hairdresser accomplishes it, the transformation is pleasing and brings a glow to the face of our completely paralyzed resident when the beautician holds up the mirror for her to see herself. We are indeed grateful for Valley Beauty Shop. It gives all of us mental and physical therapy.

Although many of us are ambulant and active most of the time, we are often forced to spend time in bed rest. When that happens, reading, television, and radio easily head the list of pastimes—though not necessarily in that order!

But it's the theater-in-the-yard just outside my window that amuses me the most. "Rascal," my little, elfish chipmunk, is the star. Rascal! That wee bit of dynamite is one of my big little bits of joy these days.

Some time ago a bird inadvertently planted a sunflower seed right up against one of my smooth metal bird-feeder poles. This sunflower grew to a height of about ten feet and made a perfect rough-surfaced ladder for Rascal to climb. From there he would hop onto the bird feeder to feast.

This morning, early, he wiggled up his rough sunflower "pole" to the whole-ear corn in the bird feeder. He filled his cheek pockets and rushed down to bury the grains of corn in my flower bed. All summer long at intervals his ingeniously planted corn sprang up among the flowers and gave the flower bed a distinctive look.

The next time I glanced out the window Mr. Rascal was sitting atop the bird feeder within reach of my hand. He sat nonchalantly for a long time with his back to me, as if to say, "I guess this will prove I am not afraid of you." It looked as if he were stationary and never intended to move. So I moved on to my next errand, which took me near the living room window.

There sat Rascal, big as life, on the arm of my lawn chair, looking right at me. His diminutiveness was accented by the outstretched acres behind him. Even the pure white three-inch chair arm spread like a concrete highway on each side of him! Soon he busied himself chasing the ground-feeding birds out of the way, since he wanted to nibble on their feed. The birds dispersed in a whir-r-r like a covey of quail scattered by a hunter's gunshot. They took haven in the luxuriant growth of purple leaves covering the flowering plum tree in front of my living room window.

Mr. Rascal is not my only animal friend. The yellow clover in the sod in front of my window entices some shy young rabbits to visit me daily. These furry creatures spark conversational exchange among the other residents, too. As two or three of us watched them from my window one day, we asked rapid-fire questions of each other.

"Why do they come to the short grass instead of staying in the field back of the building?"

"How old do you think they are?"

"Wouldn't it be fun to find their nest?"

"Do you suppose that big rabbit back of the building is their mother?"

"Aren't their ears cunning?"

"Oh, I can't bear to think of the hunters this fall."

"Opal, let's get out your guidebook on animals."

Besides all the other pleasures of our large acreage, full-grown trees and brooks bring birds to Valley Home. They feed from several bird feeders, including my two.

Enjoyable are the cardinal, mockingbird, blue jay, yellow-shafted flicker, mourning dove, redwing blackbird, and bobwhite who eat from my whole-ear corn on the ground and in the feeders. Most exciting are the song and field sparrows, slate-colored junco, Carolina chickadee and American goldfinch (wild canary) who eat the finer-ground bird feeds and are a bird-watcher's delight. The killdeer, meadowlark, crow, and robin like to strut on the blacktop and in the sod in front of my apartment. Lying on my chaise lounge, I watch the flight of nighthawks, tree swallows, purple martins, and chimney swifts—a most relaxing pastime.

One ruby-throated hummingbird produced hours of free entertainment just for me. Hovering in midair, his wings beat so fast I could hear their humming through the screened window. There he lingered, his long, curved bill in the tubes of my touch-me-not flowers.

Another time an American goldfinch put on an acrobatic act for me. After finding the huge seed-laden head of my sunflower, he was so wild with joy he acted as if he were inebriated. He flew into the sunflower head, ate, flew around in circles, returned to eat, sat on my windowsill, ate, flew against the windowpane, and repeated this routine over and over again. (Please, Lord, teach us all to use our eyesight so we may enjoy all these things you have given us to enjoy.)

Several bird happenings are entertaining enough to be recorded. When two male blue jays—fattened and strengthened by my nephew David's golden corn grains—stage regular cockfights, that's fun. When they perform atop the roof of one of my weathervane bird feeders, that's excitement. When one of them falls off his limited-size fight ring, that's real sport for me!

My interest in birds spreads to nature in general. Anne Frank, that gallant teen-ager of World War II, knew the therapeutic value of nature:

> The best remedy for those who are afraid, lonely, or unhappy is to go outside, somewhere where they can be quite alone with the heavens, nature, and God. Because only then does one feel that all is as it should be and that God wishes to see people happy, amidst the simple beauty of nature. As long as this exists, and it certainly always will, I know that then there will always be comfort for every sorrow, whatever the circumstances may be.

IX

"You Can't Waste a Season"

To every thing there is a season,
and a time to every purpose under the heaven.

Ecclesiastes 3:6

Lo, it is autumn, and I am enamored of the season. As this fall is slowly slipping in, I am fascinated by summer's transformation into flaming harvest colors. Emily Dickinson remembered the passing autumn as an "amethyst romance."

Some of the residents here at Valley still cling to the old, unscientific theory that Jack Frost alone produces the mystic alchemy that turns green trees to gold, yellow, orange, russet, and burgundy. Just to imagine Jack Frost in his pixie cap pirouetting from leaf to leaf with his palette and brush could stifle all desire to recall the mundane facts of science.

Oh, I know that mysterious dark green chlorophyll has something to do with the changing of the color and the falling of the leaves. I remember that the other colors are always present in the leaves, and that only when the chlorophyll disappears can the rich autumn carotene colors show. And I know that the length of the days and the amount of rainfall and the soil and the temperature all affect the perfect timing of this annual phenomenon.

Yet for me it is comforting to know that God, the Great Intelligence, keeps persistent order in the universe. It is he who consistently brings the seasons in proper sequence. I also know it is he who changes the young, globe-shaped trees in front of our building from living emeralds to large, irregular-cut rubies, garnets, topazes, fire opals, even amethysts that sparkle in the harvest moonlight.

Autumn plays with leaves. What pleasure I glean from watching their ethereal, rhythmic floating to the ground.

The fact that I am a bit daft about autumn leaves was singularly pointed out to me this morning. I saw in large headlines in our local paper, "LEAF COLLECTION SCHEDULED." I was impressed with the fine publicity our local Aullwood Audubon Center achieves! So I assumed they were having another exciting class in nature study and on my favorite subject, "Autumn Leaves." Even if I could not go to it, I might read about it.

Then I read the small print: "City crews will begin their annual street leaf collection . . . the leaves are to be piled . . . no sticks, stones, or other debris. . . ."

I am so sorry all our residents don't enjoy the seasonal changes. You can spend many enjoyable hours at this pastime. Some people have never enjoyed nature. Some are even amused at the ecstatic joy I get from sunsets, clouds, and the ever-changing weather at Valley.

I appreciate all the elements—even storms, thunder and lightning. Weather changes never seem common to me. Grass jeweled with dew, roofs painted with frost, blossoms jostled and tossed by the wind: they cost nothing. And they are the things I enjoy most.

I have had a few disappointments this autumn. For one thing, I sprayed my apartment too soon and too thoroughly. I have no cricket! Over at Glenside I used to allow one or two crickets to stay in Ye Olde Buggy Shoppe. They disappeared in the knotty pine closets that lined three sides of the garage. I enjoyed their chirping as Laurel and I sat before the sprightly burning fire in the buggy shoppe fireplace.

Last year I had a cricket here in my apartment. I couldn't find it, but I could hear it. (Well, maybe I didn't look very hard.)

I also missed the wild geese flying south from Canada in their V-formations. I have just not been out riding in the right area at the opportune time.

I did get to watch the nighthawks as they rallied their kin and skirted the sky over Valley night after night, sketching fantastic patterns as they flew. The sky is so lonesome without them now.

I also saw a few straggling monarch butterflies headed jaggedly southward, but not in the profusion of other years. I thrill when I think they are on their way to spend the winter as far south as Mexico. I cannot imagine so frail a creature flying such a distance.

Weather changes can help pass time even for those who are relatively inactive. I was so busy with this writing that I did not get to fully enjoy the early October morning fogs and mists as I have other years. We did not have as many mornings of such impenetrable fog at Glenside. Here I often cannot see out to the highway.

How eerie and paintable are the ever-rising, swirling mists. Our six Early American wrought iron lanterns, high up in the air on their extremely tall poles, add an artistic touch to the picturesque tableau. They remain lighted as long as the fog stays with us. The lack of sound is like a cathedral hush.

Once autumn leaves us, the bare deciduous trees on our acreage will enchant us with their striking beauty. Their gnarly, naked limbs make black silhouettes against the bleak winter skies.

A lone crow, looking a bit sinister, will flap and caw his way from oak to sycamore, never venturing near our building.

How the pristine snow will shimmer as it piles up on the bare limbs and weights down the branches and twigs. This sparkling will vary with the angle of the slanting rays of the sun. Those residents who go early to the dining room for breakfast will likely be treated to the greatest beauty. For it is those slanting rays of sun that cause the snow to be so ephemeral and steal away so quietly.

My favorite time to enjoy the snow is at night. I look out my big picture windows and watch it glisten. How could I be lonely in my apartment when the man in the moon is with me, scanning the snow from his home in the star-studded sky? I love to pull a chair up to my window at night and just sit sentiently meditating and gazing wistfully at the moon and stars. They, too, change positions with the seasons.

We enjoy the snowdrifts outside the dining room windows. The concrete platform of the patio causes the drifts to back up, layer, and ripple like sand dunes. I remember the aides pushing the wheelchair patients up to the windows last winter so they could see this miniature phenomenon.

As the thermometer fluctuates outdoors, Jack Frost may paint stars and unbelievable varieties of geometric snowflake designs on the inside of some of our windowpanes. Full well we know that this dormant stage holds the promise of spring. Then through our small-paned windows, we behold the coming of little buds. Later they burst into earlike leaves. Many of these strong, giantlike trees will bring forth dainty flowerets on their once-bare twigs. This is the time to reach for binoculars to view their intricate beauty better.

All summer long these same trees furnish relaxing, deep shade as their billowy, green tops sway with the breezes. In the summer we can watch the purple martins skittering around their well-built apartment house and study deserted bird nests. Only in summer can we enjoy sitting outdoors every day well into the evening. Then autumn rolls around again to repeat the ever-revolving circle of the seasons.

As Hal Borland quotes his farmer friend in *Homeland:* "You can't waste a season."

And, for some of us, autumn will not come again.

. . .

X

No Time for
Basket Weaving

"Preserve me from the occupational
therapist, God. She means well but
I am too busy to make baskets."
—Alise Maclay, *Green Winter*

"Are you busy?" the staff member asked as she
came into my room.

Perhaps! I was taking oxygen, watching TV, and
mending a loose jacket hem. Just then, for good
measure, a nurse came in to take my blood pressure
and pulse, and the telephone rang. How much
busier could I get?

In one book on nursing and retirement homes, I
learned that at a number of homes residents are
coerced into scheduled activities. At Valley we are

invited, encouraged, and made to feel welcome, but most certainly not coerced.

Valley provides such equipment as shuffleboard, two bicycle-type exercisers, puzzles, horseshoes, dominoes, traditional and Chinese checkers, books, two TVs, an organ, a piano, and baseball equipment. Doesn't that sound like the making of a wild life?

We have a paid activity director who plans programs, crafts, field trips, parties, and picnics. A number of residents enjoy these activities.

One of the finest things the director has accomplished is getting the people to talk—even those who are shy and confused. She comes into the group with a list of questions.

"Tell us about your first school."

"What kind of pets did you have when you were a child?"

"What games did you play when you were young?"

That last question recalls my childhood recreation when, as a tomboyish little six-year-old, my interest in "crawdads" (crayfish) was very important to me. Our old brick Colonial stood at the top of a gentle knoll overlooking a lively, stone-filled brook. I waded barefoot into the babbling water, overturned the stones, caught the hiding minnows and crawdads and ran swiftly up the hill with them.

I could enjoy them at open view in the little pools I made with bricks and sunbaked mud plaster. This I did during my relief hours after herding cattle along the grass-bordered, country dirt road. Just think! I have lived to see that rural road become a highly traveled, blacktopped highway—a main link to the Dayton airport.

At both ends of life, minnows and crayfish delight me. When young, I enjoyed them with much activity and excitement. Now old, I stand still and study their habits and life cycle . . . and reminisce.

This has been the best therapy I have seen at Valley. Memory pictures are something I never had time to indulge in before I came here. Memories can be a blessing to nursing-home residents. They can heal sorrows and soothe loneliness. I presume that is why older persons dwell on the past. It's fun. But I wouldn't ever want to substitute the present or the future for it. No, never!

Of course, an important part of any group activity is fellowship, especially those residents who do not often get away from the home and have few visitors and even fewer hobbies.

This is certainly not one of my problems! I have just three main problems: a rebellious, failing heart; only twenty-four hours in one day; and too many hobbies and interests.

Every day I enjoy, even relish, the many hobbies I've started over the years. Interests from our earlier years grow along with us as we grow older! Recently I have been delighting in two totally different pastimes: polishing some of my poems with the hope that they may find their place with the few already published, and updating the genealogies of the Hoovers and Younts, relatives of my late husband. When I am busy, I am happy!

Several women crochet and knit. There are gorgeous, brilliantly colored afghans in modish designs draped over numerous beds and wheelchairs. A wheelchair patient knitted them. Bea, who relied on a walker before she died, crocheted roses by the dozen and made them "grow" with artificial stems and leaves. Jane, in her upper eighties, has for the first time taken up painting with amazing results and delight.

Amy cleverly plans theoretical trips by means of travel literature, the only way she can now continue her many travels of bygone days. The walls in her room are decorated with the varied collection of pretty paper place mats used on our dining-room tables at Valley.

Mae, a ninety-nine-year-old lady with an exceptionally fine mind, sits at her desk, hour after hour, day after day, writing notes to relatives, friends, and acquaintances. She is meticulous in her effort to have every word correctly used. She still enjoys reading, with the help of large print and a magnifying glass. Her Bible is her favorite. This nonagenarian still appreciates the finer things in music and programming, and seldom misses a scheduled event.

Arts and crafts originate in the activity room, where there is even an electric range at our disposal. Here some of the women bake cookies and pies. Once they even made pickles! Why? Because some of the ladies, and even a man or two, have an insatiable yen to cook. It is not the easiest thing in the world to cook in your own kitchen one day and find yourself eating institutional food with a group of strangers the next. A person who has been a truly successful cook finds it extremely difficult to adjust, so the range meets a real need.

For the men the tools in a heated workshop in the three-car garage meet another need. They winter and care for geraniums, poinsettias, and other plants in that workshop. Frank Rifner, one of our ninety-four-year-olds, assembled a precut grandfather-clock kit and donated the beautiful finished clock to our pleasant dining room. It was he who bought our martin house, pole, and glorious six-by-eight-foot flag of the United States. Ladies from one of the churches come to mend and sew for the residents; Frank bought them a new sewing machine. Surely, giving for the happiness of others is a most enjoyable and rewarding way to invest your time.

One of the most fascinating pastimes for several of our men is to straw-boss any workmen who come to put in a new sewer, do carpenter work, or paint a new cottage—any job, in fact, that needs expert advice and light conversation! Then, as they lean on their canes, there is always the post-mortem to discuss how it should have been done! Many times one of them has come to me to explain the mistakes that their self-appointed committee observed.

Several other residents have their own little flower beds to admire and criticize. Our noisy Hungarian, Janos, whose frolicking with children sometimes bewilders my guests, grows luscious roses and other varicolored flowers along the concrete walks leading to the fountain.

Amy, a ninety-seven-year-old retired nurse, likes to dig in the soil and plant fruit and nut tree seeds and watch them develop. After much travail and three years' watchful care, she now has a peach tree several feet high outside her window. Potting and repotting flowers in her bathtub fills her windowsill with plants.

Outside my window a husky, persistent milkweed grows. Before it blooms, its leaves and general appearance resemble those of a rubber plant. All parts of the plant contain a milky juice called latex that gives it its name. Milkweeds are stout-stemmed plants that grow two feet or more tall.

But not mine. Until recently, Art, my farmer friend at Valley, pulled them before they could grow that tall.

"I never did like weeds!" he muttered as he pulled them.

"What practical farmer does?" I asked. "But I would really like the pleasure of seeing their broad pinkish flower clusters, Art. I promise not to let the seeds get away."

I was eager to see the exotic paisley-patterned seed pods and the ebony seeds and the fluffy white parachutes the seeds sail on in the wind.

Perhaps it's my dear little chipmunk, Rascal, that brings the fluff on seeds from elsewhere to line his nest. Rascal has entrance holes in my flower bed, so I may always have milkweed seedlings.

The next time Art trimmed my evergreens, he left

my milkweed intact. How very skillfully he did the trimming, and how willingly!

How could I have doubted that Art would stifle his agricultural instincts and suffer the milkweed to mature once he knew I had my heart set on seeing the seedpod develop? How could I have doubted, when I knew Art loves and cultivates flowers, too? After all, both of us are farmers and nature lovers at heart.

Unlike so many farmers in the Miami Valley who have just been able to eke out a living the last half century, Art was a successful dairy farmer and had raised some prize Holstein cows.

Art's large vegetable garden is as lovely to the discerning eye as his flowers. In season he keeps the home supplied with onions, carrots, tomatoes, turnips, squash, and pumpkins. This he does entirely without mechanized tools. When I asked an aide about the tools he uses, she first mentioned his hands. Of course he has a spade, rake, hand plow, and wheelbarrow—all the ordinary hand tools.

Art's health at ninety-three seems to be better than that of the rest of us, most of whom are many years his junior. He even makes occasional trips to his nephew's farm where he still does very hard physical labor.

Like the rest of us who work so diligently with our plants, Art has little time for contrived activities and basket weaving. Some of us just grow a tomato plant or two, but our enthusiasm waxes so great anyone hearing us discuss our agrarian activities would think we were managing a ranch!

XI

Grumbles, Gripes, and Gossips

One ninety-one-year-old man and his eighty-seven-year-old Valley sweetheart sat holding hands on the settee in our Fireplace Lounge. Occasionally he bent his arthritic self over to give her a peck on the cheek when he thought no one was looking.

Elizabeth wore the habit of the plain people, and William was once heard to say, "Elizabeth, I wish you would dress just a leettle more up-ter-date. Then I could see more of you!"

To a group of gossip-hungry elderly folk, that was titillating manna. Our overactive grapevine went into instant action! I was about the fifth branch down the arbor. This kind of inquisitiveness (a polite word for nosiness) helps make the hours go by.

The results lead to that pastime known as gossip—usually a holier-than-thou type! It sometimes even leads to sessions of complaints about Valley Home. (No, we are not perfect here; we are still human.) It also leads to an exchange of aches . pains . . . medicines . . . doctors . . . nurses . . . and even personalities among the residents.

Valley once had a maintenance man who was a giant physically and had a booming voice to match his size. Every so often he still returns to pay short visits to us individually or in groups. On one such occasion I was in the shower, and we did not get to chat.

Some months later Mac returned to make another call on us. As I approached the group in the hall in my motorized wheelchair, Mac cheerfully called out to me in a loud voice.

"Hey, Opal! I'm sure glad you're not in the shower, like the last time when I called on you!"

Naturally *I* understood what he meant. The puzzled looks on the faces of the other residents in the foyer distinctly and unquestionably asked, "What?!"

Although sometimes traumatic, it is also often funny when Ada, who is hard-of-hearing, misunderstands what one of us says. The redeeming thing about it is that no one laughs harder than she does. One day I used the word "hydrodiuril"—a medicine—in a sentence. "Who did you say dyed her hair?" Ada seriously queried.

It is not always a case of being hard-of-hearing. Often it is a matter of not paying careful attention, and then repeating what we *thought* we heard.

It was one of those gray shut-in days and some

residents were already quietly aware that Janos was on one of his emotional sprees. Ken, Valley's ever-faithful handyman, was talking to our aide, Valerie.

"Something Janos said really hit me," Ken remarked.

Valerie is afraid of the giant Janos. His relationship toward her has not always been too friendly. It was easy for her to visualize big Janos towering over little Ken as he hit him. It was not long until the many tendrils of the legendary grapevine had spread the now-enlarged story throughout our building: "Watch out for Janos! He hit Ken this morning. He is dangerous!"

A game that was once played at parties demonstrates the way gossip and misunderstanding get started. One person whispers a statement to another, who passes the words on to the next person. After everyone receives the message, the last member states aloud what he thought he heard. Often it barely resembles the message with which the game started.

But not all our conversation is gossip. Some very grave world problems are solved in quiet talks and louder discussions within these walls. I do not believe in eavesdropping but, please forgive me, I love to listen to "If I were president, I would. . . ." Nor can I resist listening when the discussion is about the propriety of the presence of the stalk of corn the birds planted in my flower bed.

Even the growing of sunflowers at the front of the building is questioned. Such good food for conversation! One very correct old lady was heard to say,

"Sunflowers should be planted in gardens to the rear." She should have told that to the birds!

The laundry room is another place where the atmosphere is perfect for cultivating conversation and complaints. It's not for women only, either! Some of the men help their wives with the clothes, and sometimes they even do it entirely by themselves! They even help with the ironing.

In the first few months after Valley's opening it was sometimes worth a walk to our little laundry room just to see what aides could accomplish with modern equipment. The array of shrunken, warped sweaters seemed to be the most spectacular exhibit. However, wool socks, shaped like almost anything but feet, could also have taken a prize.

Our Laundromat also had another weird capability. It could shrivel beyond recognition pajamas guaranteed by a reliable firm not to shrink more than one percent. I do not know the exact percentage our Laundromat achieved; I do know those pajamas looked like narrow-legged gaucho pants when I donned them.

My sister insists today's textiles are indeed colorfast. She cannot understand my skepticism. She has not seen our so-called colorfast pajamas turn from brilliant, cheery golds and blues to anemic, uninspiring colors. Such alchemy!

One morning I opened my door to see two old codgers looking at my doorknob in wonder. Bet their wives never wore an all-in-one bra-and-girdle combination like the one the night aide had hung on my doorknob!

Later, at the dining room table, our head nurse used the stethoscope on my chest to get an exact pulse beat and to note the changes in my heart. She had a strange, puzzled look on her face. She had hit something as hard as a rock and as big as her fist. I knew it was my foam, latex-padded bra, but I couldn't discuss it with her then and there. One nurse's aide had not yet learned how to use the laundry equipment, and she had washed it in hot water and then dried it in the electric dryer on HOT! These problems in the laundry occurred during my early days here; as the staff became more aware of the idiosyncracies of our equipment, we noted that the laundry lost a bit of its newsworthiness. There were fewer shrunken sweaters and faded pajamas to grumble or laugh about.

I prefer to laugh; it's healthier! Handicapped people are usually sweet persons. But woe be unto those who do not try to be. Those who are bitter can become very negative people. If ever anyone needs to work at keeping a good disposition, it is we who must depend upon the generosity of others' good will and help.

We have one lady here who has become bitter and entirely negative in her attitude. She reads and dwells on the most negative: brutal murders, parents who abuse children severely, bizarre accounts of life in the seventies. She growls about anything "growlable."

One day I had a bouquet of fresh-flowering dogwood. The snowy white blossoms bloomed their best. She looked at it. She smelled it.

"What's the matter with it? Did it get frost-bitten?" she snapped. She pointed to the indentations that are always on each of the four bracts on each bloom, often erroneously called petals. "Don't even smell good." Looking at our neatly mowed lawn one day she snarled, "Looks all bare since they mowed it."

A song of some years ago said something like, "Color me white, Color me blue." When I look at this pretty lady, I think how very sweet she could be. The Lord endowed her with good skin, beautiful hair, and a nice figure. But I always end up thinking "Color her gray, color her drab."

Most patients in our nursing home are not too different from what they were before they came here. If they were resourceful at home, they will most likely be resourceful in finding contentment here. We are speaking of the lucid ones, of course, who are cooperative, genial, mannerly, and respectful of the rights of others. These attributes carry over from their old-home life into this new home.

XII

When Friends Become "Family"

It didn't take long after I moved to Valley to realize something about relationships. If people made friends easily in the outside world, they will probably make friends easily in an institution. When making friends in this age-group, there is one prevalent deterrent. It has to do with memory.

A person may be alert as far as the ability to assimilate facts is concerned. He may have no difficulty retaining information. But he may have difficulty expressing himself orally. One of the most common memory lapses, I have observed, is the inability to recall the names of people and places. People of all ages have this problem, I realize, but for those who live in nursing homes, it can mean being labeled "confused."

Those who live with me here at Valley have long

since learned that most of our residents are forgetful in varying degrees. One example I recall is that of my faithful friend "B.F."

B.F. often brings objects to show me. Perhaps it's a picture he's taken, or a Christmas greeting he is fashioning. Other times it is a gadget he has made. We sit together on my sofa while he shows me his treasures, but not before he carefully lays his cane down on my already well-laden coffee table.

"I have to put my cane where I can reach it," he always explains. "I just can't walk without it anymore."

About twenty-five minutes after he has returned to his room down the long hallway, a blushing B.F. comes back and knocks on my door.

"I forgot my cane again!" He grins sheepishly.

Loss of memory doesn't have to stop friendships from forming, though. Often the exchange of mutual interests builds a strong bridge to warm relationships. Little kindnesses we perform for one another strengthen the bridge until we're no longer merely friends, but "family."

Clair and Emma, his artist wife, had been living for some time in the room next door to my apartment when I moved in. They became my first real friends at Valley, where I had not known a soul. We had much in common to encourage this friendship. But Emma was soon to be taken from us. Clair was taught by self and his two educated wives. He was a mailman by vocation and a commercial photographer by avocation. He won international acclaim some years ago with his picture of the classic winding stairway of Dayton's Montgomery County Courthouse. At Valley he is now learning a new hobby, painting.

Clair and I have both been bird-watchers for years. Flowers, especially wild flowers, also attract our interest. Clair has photographed flower close-ups, which I have never attempted. Our color travel slides run close equals. We enjoy sharing the color travel movies and slides we took with our late spouses some years ago.

I am grateful for mutual interests that encourage friendships.

One of my friends is ninety-three-year-old Ray. I could paint a better picture of Ray with a brush than I can with words. I would part that snow white, immaculately clean hair straight down the center. Then I would turn the ends in on the middle of the forehead in two quarter moon-shaped flat curls, facing each other. I am not quite sure how I could get that ever-clean, scrubbed look of his skin. What could I use from my palette besides flesh pigment?

I would bend his shoulders forward quite a bit as they try to keep up with his cane. The cane must be kept out of the portrait, since Ray is a bit sensitive about using it. I would not want to paint the shaky, unsure hands, for they would admit that Ray is aging as do his halting walk, trembling voice, and hearing failure. Those hands and voice are precious to me.

Sometimes he asks if I could use some fruit or candy or cookies. A few minutes later he's at my door with his offering of love. He holds it in one hand while he grasps the handgrip railing with the other.

He apologizes for the way it is wrapped and assures me he has washed the fruit and that the lovely napkins are unused and clean. His offerings are of the highest quality—gifts from his family and friends. He apologizes over and over for taking my time.

Helping others is almost an obsession with Ray. Therefore, he enjoys pushing me to the dining room in my wheelchair. As I sit in my chair waiting, he always approaches me with his infectious grin. "Are you out of gas, again?" he asks. He greatly enjoys this bit of his own humor. The short trip is a bit wobbly and serpentine for the chair wheels! But we haven't had a wreck yet!

I'm truly fortunate to have Ray among my family of friends. Riff was like that—family. Dear Riff. We were like two kids together. We teased and kidded each other constantly with bits of nonsense.

Riff was ninety-four and had been married to the same woman seventy-two years. She became very confused some years ago, was very frail, and had become a bit exasperating. But he insisted on keeping her in the room with him rather than letting her be moved into one of the hospital rooms. He said that after living with one woman that long, one does not wish to be separated even in the same building. He carefully and jealously watched over her.

Riff was a superb storyteller with jokes and stories galore up his sleeve. One day he was pushing me back to my apartment, balancing himself by holding on to my wheelchair. I was carrying his cane on my lap.

"Opal, I have a cute story to tell you," he chuckled. "John was pushing Mary down the street to her house. She was in her wheelchair. After they had gone some distance, he thought he heard Mary say, 'John, you're passionate.'

" Oh, no, I'm not, Mary.'

"But every few houses Mary insisted, 'John, you *are* passionate!'

"By now John was irritable when he said, 'No, I am not!' But she insisted that he was.

"John could not hear well, but he really could see better than Mary. He began to think that they ought to be about there. He looked around.

" 'My gosh! Mary, we've passed your house. I'll have to push you back uphill.'

"Undisturbed, but in a louder voice, Mary retorted, 'I've kept saying all along that you're passin' it, and you kept saying you weren't!' "

It was a familiar sight at Valley to see Riff standing in the corridor sharing his fun with another resident. His jokes and stories, founded upon his keen sense of humor, were good for the morale of Valley Home residents. He turned sour countenances into smiling ones.

One evening Riff came to my door in tears. "May I come in, please? I'm so blue I just have to talk to someone."

He poured out his troubles to me. No one had visited him. No one had telephoned him. No one had written him. His eyes were failing and he could no longer read or spend time with his tools wood-working.

The younger gentleman who had regularly taken him out to eat had just undergone open-heart surgery. Riff was worried about his friend's recovery and he was also concerned that it would be a long time before they could go out to eat together again. As for himself, he was just not feeling good at all.

Then I told him about my book. "Would you like to hear some of it, Riff? You're in it, if that's all right with you."

His face radiated. "Oh, Opal, I'd be so proud." As I read to him he laughed loudly and heartily at his own jokes, and he seemed to be lighter-hearted when he said good night.

A few days later Riff quietly went to be with the Lord, and just a week later his wife Dolly joined him. They died peacefully, but not before Riff had touched my life with joy and humor and childlike mischief.

XIII

Of Minds and Medicine

It is Monday morning at Valley, and soon a nurse will be in to take my blood pressure. This they do routinely three mornings each week. Mondays are a bit different for me from the other days of the week, since I have more nursing attention. This is especially noteworthy since we are an intermediate-care facility, not a skilled nursing facility or hospital.

If I have an acute illness, my personal physician, Dr. Hammond, requests blood-pressure checks every day. The nurse who takes my blood pressure may have a second nurse give me a liver shot, but this only happens once a week.

My medicine sometimes comes on the breakfast tray. But whenever and however it comes, the nurse always takes my pulse, seven days a week, to make sure the digitalis is properly regulating my heart. All residents are also weighed at the nurses' station once each month.

Every Monday morning a laboratory technician comes to take blood out of my arm to see how long it takes my blood to clot. These tests are necessary because I have thrombophlebitis (clotting in the veins). To control this clotting, I'm given a medicine that thins my blood. The test measures the effectiveness of the medicine.

I buy all my medicines from a local pharmacist, although we may purchase them from anywhere we want. Dr. Hammond writes the prescriptions. The nurses at Valley keep track of my medicine and reorder whenever necessary. All I have to do is take the medicine according to directions and pay the itemized bill—which averages well above eighty dollars monthly!

I send my health insurance company a complete record of each individual purchase, including the nature of my illness, the prescription number, the date of purchase, the name of my pharmacist, my doctor's name, and the price of the drug. The insurance company reimburses a percentage of the monthly cost for prescription medicines.

A podiatrist comes to my room the first Thursday of every month to care for my feet. This is an expense not covered by Valley. There is no provision for dental or optometric services, either.

Something my nephew Ron and his lovely wife, Peg, gave me challenges me to rebuke any dismay I could feel about all the medical attention I get. It's a framed picture of their children, Brian and Amy. It makes me both happy and sad.

I did not get to see their brave Brian much the last year he lived. He was battling cancer and was in and out of the Children's Medical Center. What a legacy of mature acceptance and courage he left me!

When a resident here tells me how much she suffers with an I.V. (intravenous) needle in her arm for "three whole hours," I remember how Brian learned to get down on the floor and play by the hour with that I.V. in his arm, how he asked for the I.V. for feeding when he was too sick to eat, how he asked to be taken back to the hospital when his lungs started to fill up with fluid again. Four years old! When I have to face the almost impossible, I pray to God to grant me Brian's mature courage.

It's facing change that seems most difficult to some people. But age means changes that involve the whole person, not simply wrinkling skin and deteriorating bodily functions. Sometimes it means confusion, especially if high-powered drugs are needed for one reason or another. Often, perfectly sane people can become confused after the dispensation of these drugs.

That was the case late one night recently. There was poor little Eva, streaking down the public hallway in her birthday suit. Instead of entering her bathroom door, she had exited through her hall door. I hurried to lead her back to her room, praying silently that no one else would see the usually refined and decorous Eva in this state.

It must have been the recognition of me that brought her memory back. She apologized frantically as she tried to make two hands cover more than two spots until she was safely in her own room! All the time she was saying, "Oh, Opal, *excuse me*, *excuse me*." *How gladly* I excused her!

One evening during chapel, my own pastor, Dr. William Schram, gave a brilliant word picture of his trip to Russia. I had invited a number of my fellow churchmembers to my apartment for a bit of sociability and refreshments after the program. Tucky crashed the party—repeatedly.

"Opal!" she insisted. "Please come to my room and help me!" A nurse's aide took her back to her room, but a few minutes later Tucky burst through my doorway again.

"Opal! You're good to everybody else. I can't understand why you won't help me take care of the baby!" This time the administrator returned Tucky, but it wasn't long before she was back.

"Opal! You know I can't manage the baby by myself!"

This time my party simply broke up. Oh, why did she come? I was furious! Why didn't they sedate her? I knew there must be a reason.

I am happy to report that Tucky's mind is now stable, and I find her a delight. High-powered drugs had apparently confused her mind, as often happens after hospitalization.

We have two older women here at Valley whose minds, for whatever reason, have failed. They live together in a double room. Dessa sometimes screams at the top of her voice. (I have read in numerous books on nursing homes that at least one such individual case is par for the course at institutions for the aged.) Naomi, the other lady, had been a schoolteacher. She is quiet and dignified. In our earlier years, before she became confused, we enjoyed our friendship. We had much in common.

Our young housekeeper, Lila, who works here to earn money toward college expenses, enjoys studying individual residents for her psychology class. She has observed the surviving schoolteacher attitudes, gestures, and speech of Naomi. (Schoolteachers have long been stereotyped. "You can tell she is a schoolteacher." "She has all the looks of a schoolteacher." "Acts just like a schoolteacher." I can remember when I first came to Valley I actually resented it when someone remarked, "Oh, that's the schoolteacher in you cropping out.")

One day Lila was cleaning near Naomi's bed when Dessa let out a whale of a scream. Naomi straightened to a dignified position and shook her hand with her finger pointed in true schoolteacher fashion at Dessa. "Now, don't you ever do that again!" she declared.

Encouraged by this negative command, Dessa screamed louder than ever. Naomi sharply reprimanded, "I told you not to do that again." With that she whammed Lila, the housekeeper, on top of the head several times! The schoolteacher had met the call of duty. Discipline had been administered—even though the object was not the right one!

Yes, of course, we have patients who answer to Webster's description of senility: "suffering loss or weakness of bodily health and strength and mental

113

powers, as so often occurs in old age." Notice Webster put loss of mental powers last and he did not say old age was the cause.

And just because a person is aged and infirm does not mean he is unable to reason. One of our nurses learned that in an embarassing way one evening.

My ninety-five-year-old mother came to live at Valley during the last several months of her life. One night in Mother's first week here she had a nightmare—a horrible dream! In telling me about it the next morning, she said that after she woke up there was a nurse with two of her aides sitting on her sofa for a long, long time.

It troubled her that they were laughing and giggling, for she thought it must have been about her experience. But what really worried her was how they would ever get their work done!

One of the aides came to gossip with me about it the next night. I was eager to tell her that Mother had already told me all about the nightmare experience! When I informed the aide that their ninety-five-year-old patient was still concerned about the three of them visiting in her room so long, she was genuinely shocked. The women had not realized that Mother could see or hear them since she was legally blind and somewhat deaf.

In September 1979 in a special report on aging, the National Institute of Health noted that "senility is not an inevitable consequence of growing old; in fact, it is not even a disease. . . . Rather, senility is a word commonly used to describe a large number of conditions. . . ."

Symptoms of senility include confusion, loss of memory, stupor, delirium, hyperactivity, self-centered worry or focus on self (even to unusual, extreme worries about bowel habits). What is called senility alters not only thought and memory but also appetite, walking, sitting, sleeping, and other bodily functions.

However, modern medicine has concluded that aging alone is not responsible for loss of mental ability. In fact, research suggests that there are more than twenty other causes, including accidents to the spine, head injuries, or depression. Senility's symptoms may also be caused by such diseases as acute thyroid deficiency, severe illness with high fever, blood vessel spasms of the brain.

Arteriosclerosis, intense worry, imbalance of electrolytes, dehydration, wrong or too much medicine, extreme fatigue, heart failure, pneumonia, and strokes. Some researchers even include lack of sunshine (vitamin D absorption), malnutrition, anemia, brain disease, infections, and frustration.

When you know someone who shows one or more of these symptoms of senility, you should find a physician with keen diagnostic ability. He should be familiar with geriatrics and know that old age alone may not be responsible. He should check to be sure there are no other causes for the symptoms.

When an individual recognizes his tendency to get confused, he will often aggravate the problem by worrying about it. This is another reason why early treatment is important.

A member of the family should go with the person

to make sure the doctor knows the whole story. Before deciding to put that person in a nursing home, his family should be sure he has gone to a hospital known for its geriatic work and gotten all the appropriate examinations.

As we get older, of course, we all suffer from loss of bodily health and strength. None of us has the mental agility we had when we were younger. In any nursing home "family" there will be those who have real problems with senility.

We are, however, changing the way we respond to the aging mind with chronic or acute brain impairment. Once these unfortunate people were pronounced incurable and sent to an asylum to worsen daily. They were separated from all family members and friends. They were deserted.

I'm grateful I took time to study nursing-home facilities so I could find one where staff members know how to find the real person behind the befuddled mind.

Valley is an intermediate care center. It is not even an advanced nursing home, let alone a hospital. Our staff is not hired to do mental therapy, nor do we have special equipment for it. All we have is the general run of games and bicycle exercisers, though we also have some nurses with reality orientation training and laboratories from which technicians come regularly to administer those tests the doctors request.

But even more important for the person who is mentally impaired, our nursing staff members are competent and genuinely concerned. The "senile" person usually responds quickly to kindness, love, understanding, and patience. He wants someone to talk with. He may tell wild tales. But here at Valley the staff and many of the residents try to help by listening patiently.

A ninety-three-year-old woman may tell you, "My mother is coming to see me tonight." Another may continually put on her coat and pick up her handbag ready to go home. Oh, how they want to go home—and sometimes they try it!

Occasionally, it is even possible to reason with some of them. "Now, Katherine, you are— what?—eighty-five years old? You know your mother would be over a hundred. She has gone to heaven." Or "None of us are going back to our old homes tonight. This is our home now. We all live here day and night together. We are one big family." It may help for a time, but is usually soon forgotten.

Our staff tries to encourage the interests of the patient. John may like to paint or putter with clay. Mary may like to read. Those who are physically able are taken to programs, movies, and religious services with the hope that this type of involvement with others will help them. Often I see an aide talking and talking as she walks a patient. An effort is made to keep everyone mobile. Activity classes keep hands busy. A well-organized group of church volunteers take turns visiting and conversing. The home encourages family members to visit as often as possible. Patients who are able are encouraged to participate in physical exercise classes. Most of them like music, too. And to encourage a sense of belonging, the staff brings together "buddies" who have similar interests.

All this exposure, it is hoped, helps to keep the senile individual diverted and more relaxed. Sometimes he may be so unhappy, and even violent, that the doctor orders sedatives and sleeping pills. Occasionally, senile patients have to be confined to bed or geriatric chairs. The nurses put them in chairs near the nurses' station where they can be watched carefully while they watch television.

In most cases those given this care improve, sometimes dramatically. We have had no "complete recoveries" at Valley, although one patient returned to normal when doctors took her off the medicine she had been given at the hospital. Our administrator says he doesn't know anyone who is senile who has completely recovered.

Yet both of us witnessed the miraculous transformation of one individual. Gwen, an eighty-three-year-old woman who had suffered two severe strokes, was brought here to die. She seemed wild, mean, defiant, unappreciative, ill-mannered—all the undesirable traits you can think of. We all wondered how she could have had the highly successful career she enjoyed in her profession in her younger years.

She was in a single room across the hall from mine. If I left my door open I got the full benefit of her thunderous voice. She certainly did not have the oxygen shortage I suffer!

All up and down the hallway I could hear her reiterating "One-one-one" or "Seven-seven-

seven" in bellowing shouts, or giving a long, loud, weird-sounding wail. Occasionally there would be an outburst of loud talking—to herself! I greatly resented her being here. As is my normal habit, I was very vocal about her presence.

"This is no place for Gwen," I told one of the nurses. "She should be in a mental care center where they are prepared to care for her and possibly improve her condition." On and on I voiced my objections, for I knew that Valley did not have to keep her here.

"But, Opal," the nurse replied, "we must accept Gwen for what she is. We can't stereotype her. Her main trouble is frustration. She was all alone in a big house before she came here. I suppose that when she realized she was becoming confused she was terrified.

"Maybe she feels she should not have lived so long and fears the road ahead. Perhaps if she sees that somebody cares and wants to help her, she'll begin to help herself."

Later, in my quiet times with God, I realized that my attitude didn't please him. It wasn't easy for me, but I went to visit Gwen with a gift of a perfect rosebud in a vase. She was in one of her word-repeating predicaments, but she knew what she was doing.

"Gwen," I said softly, "I want to be your friend."

Her dour expression did not change, but she nodded. I started to set the bud vase down on the tray of her "geri-chair."

"Three—three—three!" she roared, pointing to a

table in the corner of the room. She had already thrown trays across her room a number of times, and since I had to walk in front of her I was a bit fearful. What if I became her next victim?

She continued to repeat her loud, raucous yelling. "And—And—And!" Suddenly she broke in just long enough to look at me and force out the words, "Can't stop."

"That's all right," I told her. "I understand. I'll come and visit you again."

Over the next weeks I continued to visit Gwen, and I felt I was gaining some ground. The staff's determination to meet the challenge and do something for Gwen encouraged me. It was a special challenge to help this little lady who had once been so attractive and brilliant.

As the months went on, Gwen relaxed. She started to talk normally, at first only occasionally but then more and more often. She began to read. She wanted to be dressed properly, and she took care of her own personal hygiene. She became interested in and proud of her family, and even called them on the telephone. She began to write letters and to crochet. She asked for family pictures to decorate her room, and she insisted on running her own wheelchair to take care of herself. Above all, she became appreciative and polite.

The therapy of love had accomplished an unusual transformation!

XIV

Stop the Bookmobile! Turn on the TV!

It is not true that we have
only one life to live; if
we can read, we can live as
many more lives and as many
kinds of lives as we wish.
—S. I. Hayakawa

Sometime during the afternoon every other Monday, a day brightener appears. With unfailing regularity, the Dayton-Montgomery County Public Library bookmobile makes its stop, laden with the books our residents have requested.

Reading is almost as popular a pastime as television at Valley. Many of the residents use a reading glass. Since this is a church-oriented home, the Bible leads the list of requests, with Christian books and magazines a close second.

One thing is certain, we can get all the books we

want on almost any subject we desire from the bookmobile's outstanding service. The van brings as many books as we request. When we don't know what we want, the librarian in charge of the book-mobile department, Mr. David Roach, will make selections for us.

Dave makes a point of knowing the reading tastes of everyone at Valley, including those he has never met. He's learned these preferences so well that he only needs the name to make a selection. One time a patron asked for a book on Harry Truman, but before the request came in Dave had already placed it in his bag!

He puts books in plastic drawstring bags large enough to carry as many as a dozen books. Each bag is imprinted in large black letters, "Dayton-Montgomery County Bookmobile." (This prevents residents and staff from confusing empty library bags with other service bags used at Valley.) Finally, a heavy Manila tag with the resident's name, also printed in heavy black letters, is tied to the draw-string.

Since he is in charge of services to the homebound, Dave spends every Tuesday and Fri-day selecting an average of six books for each person on his bookmobile route. He doesn't choose all our books, of course. We have the privilege of request-ing and renewing books. It is especially nice to be able to get many of the more recent publications through the bookmobile that it's almost impossible to get at any of the library buildings!

Often the deaf, as well as a few other residents,

cannot order books for themselves. Others are unable (and sometimes unwilling) to order for themselves. To help them, I have the bookmobile department send large books of pictures—animals, flowers, birds, travel, and the like—in my name. I pass these along, and I've found many appreciate and enjoy looking at them.

The bookmobile also brings long-playing records and cassette tapes as well as books. Dave knows I like classical records, so classics are what I get. The tapes offer more variety: music, travel, poetry, biographies, history.

One of our college-educated men is legally blind and somewhat deaf. He takes full advantage of the Talking Book Service of the Library of Congress. In this way he keeps entertained and informed—and happy. He uses earphones, so he disturbs no one.

I once had the government's talking-book record player. But I changed to tapes because the tape recorder is small enough (7'' x 7''x 2½'' deep) to put on my bedside table where I can reach it anytime I want. Unfortunately, there are a lot more phonograph talking-book records than tapes. I hope that will soon change.

You can help the resident of any nursing home get a cassette tape player or a record player free of charge through the Library of Congress. Write:

> Library of Congress
> National Library Service
> for the Blind and Physically Handicapped
> Washington, DC 20542

The Library of Congress Reading Book Service is available to nursing-home residents in all states. Once a person receives the machine, he will also be sent lists of the titles of the talking books (records or cassette tapes) available. These lists are extensive and should meet anyone's needs. You can make all these transactions by mail, free of charge. If a machine needs repair, it may be put back in the case it came in and returned by mail, so it's important to save the mailing case for future use.

Several of our women spend a lot of time with various types of puzzles—especially crossword puzzles. This pastime often sends them to the dictionary and other books for information and is in addition a fine antidote for loneliness.

Learning of any kind is. That's why for four years, I arranged programs for the residents every Tuesday night—not just the "busy-work" type of program that so often comes to nursing homes. We didn't get any kind of grant for these programs. But through my friends' acquaintances and my own, I was able to get the kind of talent that usually appeared only for a fee.

There were soloists from Dayton's Philharmonic Orchestra and the entire Dayton Music Appreciation Group (one of Dayton's oldest and finest musical groups). We had illustrated lectures from one of the four National Audubon Centers in the United States, and entertainment from the Dayton Banjo Club and puppet groups. Everyone seemed to enjoy the programs and learn a lot from them.

A number of the residents who cannot see well

enough to read watch television. Most of the residents select what they watch more carefully than you might think. They are very interested in what our presidents and other government representatives and nationally known religious leaders have to say.

It isn't often I let TV keep me from other activities. But one day I glued myself to it. I was relieved that no one came to my apartment that day! That way I didn't have to turn my TV off. I didn't want to miss a minute of the festivities. This, you see, was America's birthday party on TV—the glorious Fourth of July bicentennial celebration.

Always a flag-waver, I let my emotions run in high gear, unchecked. I couldn't take my eyes off the beautifully portrayed programs and parades. Celebrations were televised from Washington, Philadelphia, New York, Miami Beach, San Francisco, France—all over the world, in fact. Even England, the country from which our independence was won, got into the act with a show hosted by Alistair Cooke. Big Ben, the famous British timekeeper, chimed long and steadily.

I accepted the invitation the television stations issued to citizens all over the United States and Europe to join in ringing bells simultaneously at two o'clock. I could see and hear many world-famous bells as I lounged on my rolled-up electric hospital bed and rang *my* Pakistani brass bell and my cowbell from the farm.

Chimes pealed from cathedrals and courthouses, from churches and California missions, joining me

125

in proud celebration of my country's birth and its subsequent growth and development. There will be other Independence Day celebrations; but July 4, 1976, will outrank any I will ever be part of. The bicentennial blazed into my heart and mind the prayer that the United States will always be a leader in the quest for universal justice and world peace.

I was relieved to remember that the nurses do not come to my room to take my blood pressure on Sunday. I was further pleased that no one caught me saluting the flag as I sat there in bed. Sometimes you have to watch what you do when you live in a nursing home. They could think I was a bit confused. (Maybe I am, but I just don't want anyone to know it!)

Good television programs help keep nursing-home residents in touch with the outside world. Some of us find time on Sunday morning for programs such as "Call the Doctor," "Meet the Press," and "Face the Nation," which are indeed educational. I often turn to my favorite public television station for an evening of symphony orchestra music. Then for contrast I enjoy arguing with William F. Buckley, Jr., on "Firing Line."

Wile animal and general nature programs such as the National Geographic specials are also headliners at Valley. So, of course, are game and talk shows. The variety of television programming stimulates our thinking and keeps us from becoming isolated from the world outside the nursing home. We're grateful for it.

XV

"But I Thought
You Were a Methodist!"

On my lengthy list of minister acquaintances is the present pastor of my girlhood church. Recently the Reverend Forthright telephoned to thank me for a publication I had mailed him. In the course of our conversation he told me stories of his early contacts with Presbyterians, many of whom he felt were arrogant.

He unknowingly continued to emphasize this negative quality until I jokingly asked him, "Aren't you ashamed to talk about Presbyterians that way to someone who has been a Presbyterian for almost fifty years?"

"B-but," he hesitated, "I always thought you were a Methodist!"

Maybe I had once told him about the delightful class of teen-age girls I had once taught at our local Methodist church. Would he have been confused to learn about the Baptist Sunday school class I once enjoyed teaching, too!

I CHOSE TO LIVE IN A NURSING HOME

Perhaps it's because I enjoyed sharing in the fellowship of all kinds of Christians when I was young that I enjoy chapel and Bible study so much here at Valley. We have regularly scheduled chapel here on Sundays with lots of hearty hymn singing. Each Wednesday morning we have discussion and prayer, and Bible study on Thursday mornings. Since this is a church-sponsored home, these sessions are well-attended.

Jane Jennings, a woman from my home church, comes weekly with the printed program and recorded tape of the previous Sunday service. She even has time left to visit with me. We find a lot to discuss in spite of—perhaps because of—the difference in our ages. Dear little optimistic Jane with the beautiful red hair and green eyes. Just to look at her gives me a lift!

Besides the church bulletin and tape of each Sunday's services, I get by mail "Westminster Chimes," our semimonthly church news bulletin and *A. D.*, our United Presbyterian Church monthly magazine. Even though I am in this nursing home and never see the inside of my old home church, these communications and my visitors give me the feeling of still belonging.

When I play the tape of my own Westminster United Presbyterian Church service, I imagine I am sitting with Laurel in our same old pew. I can see the stained-glass windows scintillating on either side of the long sanctuary. The famous Tiffany Studios' Te Deum window behind the choir complements their blending choir robes.

I sometimes close my eyes as the full deep tones of the two Cassavant organs introduce the choir. I affirm our belief with the entire congregation. My Bible is open and ready to follow along with Pastor William Schram's invitation, "Listen to the Word." I pray the Lord's Prayer aloud with my fellow church members. I have been to church!

Each resident has his own favorite Sunday morning television service. Almost every television in the building is following what some internationally known minister or speaker has to say. I spend some Sunday mornings going from one service to another, each chosen because the speaker has something from God to share with me.

When I go to the local churches' presentation, "Church by the Side of the Road," I am exposed to many different churches scattered over the entire Miami Valley. Sometimes it's a "Catholic Mass"; sometimes it's the Baptist-oriented "Landmark Bible Class" from Cincinnati. "Catholic Mass" is broadcast from a different church each week, as is "Church by the Side of the Road." I rather enjoy watching these changes of setting and comparing the services.

"Day of Discovery" with Richard De Haan brings back memories of the old "Radio Bible Class," originated and developed by the late Dr. Martin R. De Haan, his father. This splendid TV program reaches us from Cypress Gardens, Florida, every Sunday morning.

Richard De Haan, a well-informed Bible teacher, is my kind of preacher! He offers calm, conversational Bible study, helpfully applied to present-day living, without any shouting or pressure gimmicks. I enjoy the music, and the serene beauty of Cypress Gardens (which I often enjoyed in person with my husband) adds to the serious study.

Dr. Robert Schuller stands proudly and confidently at the head of my list of preachers when he brings "The Hour of Power." I like well-planned, beautiful, thought-provoking services. "The Hour of Power" leaves me inspired and encouraged.

The hour is filled with exquisite music and engaging guests. The superb television camera work makes me feel as if I could reach out and shake hands with Dr. Schuller. I can almost smell the pleasingly arranged flowers, walk through the magnificent cathedral, and hear the water tumbling in the fountain near the well-sculptured statue of the Shepherd and his sheep. On so many religious TV programs the visual qualities are distracting. "The Hour of Power" offers the possibility thinking in the Word of God to inspire me for one more week.

One of my favorite programs is "It Is Written," with George Vandeman as the speaker. His information, which is presented earnestly in a soothing, loving voice, brings much food for thought. He talks rather than preaches, and the only time I have detected anything distinctively Seventh-Day Adventist was once when he mentioned vegetarianism!

"Dialogue," a panel discussion composed of a Roman Catholic, a Jew, a Protestant, and often a black Christian is a most enlightening program. It is not only interesting and educational, but it makes me think.

I should also mention two men I greatly admire for the Christian universities they have founded and the faith they have helped young people find—Jerry Falwell and Oral Roberts.

The main advantage I have found in traveling from church to church via television is that it gets me out of my own narrow little groove. I begin to notice similarities as well as differences.

At the same time I am more aware of the need for a variety of churches in which we can express our Christian faith according to our own personalities. Some of us like to shout! Some of us prefer the decorum of dignity and pageantry. The important thing is a biblically oriented faith in Jesus Christ.

Some of my readers may feel I am too "ecumenical," I realize. But I am grateful to be able to recognize the contribution of churches that differ quite a bit from my own. But then, I think I differ a wee bit from some Presbyterianisms, too! I think for myself, and I know the Lord loves me!

By twelve thirty, when Sunday dinner is announced, I have been informed, aroused, questioned, irritated, alerted, inspired, convinced, motivated, challenged—you name it, I've experienced it! Through these many talks I have had all the benefits of a rousing good seminar—all in one morning, all in the time it would have taken me to go to one church in person if I had been able to go.

Besides, TV offers the prerogative of turning away from one channel and tuning in a preference. I hesitate to admit it, but I have benefited much more fully, knowledge-wise, than I could ever have by attending one church service in person.

Then why shouldn't everyone do what I do? I'm not missing anything, am I?

Yes, I am! I miss very much the inspiration of fellowship with other church members. I miss the joy of working with a purpose within groups of an organized church. Much more, I miss the privilege and the benefits of being a member or a leader of one or more of those groups. That's the biggest weakness of "TV religion." It entertains and stimulates, but it can't give you the fellowship Christ wants us all to enjoy in the church.

Some nursing-home residents are still able to attend the church of their choice. I recommend that you go to a church in person as often and as long as you can. But when you can no longer do so, my way is the next best thing to being there!

XVI

"I Wonder What He Does for a Living?"

Joe, our administrator, was standing quietly behind the podium waiting for our grandfather clock to chime twelve o'clock. When it did, he would begin our daily devotional time. Most of us had already quieted down. In that hush it was easy for Joe to hear the few remarks still being made here and there—especially from the tables up front.

Out of the prevailing stillness came the audible remark, "I wonder what he does for a living?"

Now the person doing all that wondering is not entirely confused, but she is most certainly not lucid enough to understand that the man behind the pulpit was the administrator of the home she was living in! Even less could she understand what the administrator of a small nursing home like Valley does.

At that moment, of course, Joe was our chaplain. Larger homes often have full-time chaplains. Joe not

133

only leads daily devotions, he also has a weekly morning session of prayer and discussion and arranges for Sunday chapel and weekly Bible study periods.

When anyone is ill or troubled, it is Joe who, acting as chaplain, goes to the individual's room for prayer, counsel, and comfort. And when someone becomes critically ill or dies at any hour, day or night, Joe is called. Sometimes he has had to make complete funeral arrangements and estate settlements. He's even scattered the ashes of some former residents to comply with their requests. He has often taken care of a patient's Medicare and other business affairs when that person has been too ill to do for himself.

Recently a young girl applied for a job in Valley's kitchen. Joe inquired about her former job. She had worked for one of the large and well-known nursing homes in this area. Her job had been to keep the shelves in the stockroom filled for the kitchen crew. Joe had to tell her he did all that at Valley by himself!

In a small home the administrator does the marketing and purchasing for all departments: office supplies, janitorial supplies, and such kitchen supplies as utensils, appliances, dinner mats, napkins, dishes, and cutlery. He pays all the bills. He makes all the necessary trips to the bank and post office. These duties would be shared by a purchasing agent and the business administrator at a larger nursing home.

Our administrator shops not only for the needs of the home but also for individual residents for whom he buys such things as stockings, hair nets, note paper, stamps, and toothpaste. He is dedicated to keeping us happy.

I remember that one time, in order to pacify an elderly lady, Joe had to exchange one tube of toothpaste for a different size because it did not fit into her medicine cabinet the way she liked to arrange it! If a patient's diet specifies certain foods, it is Joe's responsibility to purchase it. He even takes broken dentures to the dentist and eyeglasses to the optician for repair or new lenses.

Joe is also head chauffeur here. If a resident has no other way to get to his doctor or dentist, Joe drives the Valley bus to the resident's destination.

The administrator of a small home puts help-wanted ads in the newspaper. He handles all telephone and mail communication concerning jobs. He conducts all interviews with prospective staff members. He hires and fires. His only helper in all this is a secretary-bookkeeper.

Our administrator gives all prospective residents a tour of the building and negotiates all transactions if they decide to enter. He hosts visiting dignitaries and arranges for them to eat in our attractive dining room.

The district conference of the churches that support Valley appoints a nine-member board of trustees to select and guide the administrator.

He in turn is responsible for a staff of twenty-two employees. Since we have an average of forty-seven residents, there is one staff member for every two of us. Three people handle the utilities, maintenance, and other housekeeping. There are six on the kitchen staff, and we have thirteen nurses and aides.

With a staff this size Joe doesn't have any idle time. When he's not meeting the responsibilities I've described, he's expected to spend time doing deputation work for the home. He speaks at various sponsoring churches to urge members of the congregations to help spiritually and financially, especially through provisions of wills and trust funds.

Then, of course, there are meetings. As a chaplain, Valley's administrator is a member of the local Ministerial Association that meets once a month. There is also a monthly meeting of the Administrators of Philanthropic Homes. Furthermore, all nursing-home administrators must attend twenty-one hours of seminar training in order to renew their licenses. Once a month our administrator wades the sometimes troubled waters of meetings of the board of trustees and attempts to keep its members conscious of the fact that they are supposed to be "brethren in grace."

If a person is the administrator of a small nursing home, I no longer wonder what he does for a living!

XVII

"I Brought You Something"

As a child I always delighted in little gifts from visitors. Most people can recall the pleasures of little unbirthday gifts and no-special-reason remembrances. How much more a gift means to a person who is confined to an institution, dependent upon others for almost everything.

One "gift" I treasure most is children, many of whom are learning to be kind and share with others. Often they present programs for us, and usually they bring us some small handmade gift. Sunday school classes, Scouts, Brownies, Camp Fire Girls, Pioneer Girls, and choirs all share their talents.

It's the child, I think, we miss most when we live in a nursing home. One book I read said that some homes actually refuse to allow children as visitors! I'm grateful that this is not true of Valley. Children are regarded as good therapy here.

Sometimes family members bring musical instruments to play for us. It's fun! My grandniece Laurie plays the flute; Christy brings her pint-size violin and twirls her baton. Twirling a baton in my memento-filled room may make me nervous at times, but Christy never misses! At present, their brother Harris displays his musical talent by singing for me. I think his parents might not consider investing in the drums he wants.

My only niece, Linda, brings or mails me reports and examples of school, Sunday school, and 4-H Club activities. She keeps me informed about the family's musical activity and prowess in swimming, horseback riding, skating, and track meets. This is a delight to an old auntie who cannot see them perform in person. Recently, Laurie came to report on the trip she took with her Miamisburg School Band to Georgian Bay country in Canada. From what she shared, I was able to experience her trip with her in my mind.

I enjoy painting such mental pictures. One such portrait is of my nephew Ron's wife, Peggy. She is sitting in my tall-backed rose rocker, her delicate natural blonde beauty contrasting with the dark walnut-color caning. Cuddled in her arms is little Amy. Young Brian is standing beside them, leaning his head on Peggy's shoulder. Although Brian is in heaven now, this is one Madonna painting that is indelibly painted on my memory. Time will not erase it.

Another memory portrait was framed in my picture window one day. Standing outdoors, looking in, was my brother Myron and his wife, Jo. Myron was cuddling their little sunshine-filled granddaughter Amy on the eve of her first birthday. They were all three waving hands as if generated by electricity.

Few people realize that such small, loving acts are really contributions to our health and happiness. Unless people bring children to see us, we miss out on some of life's richest experiences. How could I do without the memory of the time when Christy, at the age of three, baked the first birthday cake I had after moving into Valley? How I value the memory of the large fruit cocktail cakes Laurie and Linda repeatedly made for me. How treasured are the lovely gifts they brought me from time to time. These are tangible evidences of love and concern anyone can understand and appreciate.

But please read between the lines and catch all the more important *intangible* things that children can do for us, too. A very small favor can linger and multiply through the years. When I first came here, Myron planted a few members of the sedum plant family (hen and chickens) from Glenside around my bird-feeder pole. I would venture to say that the people who have enjoyed them since number in the hundreds.

Those chickens grew into hens and the hens "hatched" more chickens. (If you've never enjoyed this little plant, pick one up at a local nursery!) When taking plants to a retirement-home resident, take ones that will practically take care of themselves, such as any of the large family of sedums.

My other brother, Lowell, has a prize-winning garden. He and his wife, Kay, bring me weekly bouquets from the flowers that bloom there from early spring to late frost. His luxuriant roses are a special treat. I often take out several buds and send single roses in bud vases to some of our residents.

Usually, Kay has the flowers all arranged in a vase or bowl before she brings them into my room. If not, she gets a vase from my ample supply and arranges them here. Please remember, when you bring flowers to a nursing home, that it causes a bit of a problem if you bring them in and lay them down on a table or give them to an aide to take care of. Kay's way is best. Neither she nor any other of my visitors has ever bothered an aide to take care of the flowers they have brought.

Marilyn, their son David's wife, knows my diet and brings only the kind of candy she knows I can eat. Her homemade "hardtack"—I much prefer the more modern name, stained-glass candy—looks just like the panes in a cathedral. But even better, David and Marilyn bring me their five darling children. What a delight it is to hear them tell "Aunt Opal" all about their farm animals!

Kay is the only member of my family who writes me a newsy letter every week. In reference to her mail I am often reminded of the adage, "It is not only the realization thereof, but the anticipation thereof." You may want to give this double gift of realization and anticipation to someone in a nursing home.

When Kay and Lowell are traveling, I know I will

hear from them and will not have to wonder how and where they are. As do Corrinne and John, on their return they share with me the color slides they take on these trips.

When the incoming mail is delivered at Valley, I over and over again hear others bemoan the fact that they never get any. Please send letters or cards to those you know in a nursing or retirement home. They appreciate it more than most of you can imagine. If the resident is a relative of yours, he is almost certain to enjoy the family mail you receive. When you visit, why not bring it to the nursing home and share it?

One time one of my nurse friends volunteered to type the manuscript of this book (free of charge) after her baby arrived. She said she would have so much time on her hands after she quit her nursing activities here at Valley that she would welcome the typing as something to help pass her time.

I appreciated the offer. But I had helped to care for my sister and two brothers from the days they were born at our parents' farmhouse, so I knew just how much spare time Terry was going to have! After the baby was here a short time, Terry telephoned me and we had a good laugh about all the idle time she was not having.

I accidentally found a new idea for retired people recently as I was browsing through my National Retired Teachers' Association News Bulletin. In the British Isles a pen-pal organization called the Saga Club, with a membership of more than 500,000 persons over the age of sixty-five, wants to correspond with its equivalent in the United States. How I would enjoy being part of that!

If you know someone who might like to develop an international friendship, write to:

The Saga Club
98 Sandgate Road
Folkestone
Kent, England.

If the resident is well enough to carry on a correspondence, he will need stamps, letter paper, some greeting cards, and pen and pencil. He will also need either refills or replacements, since most nursing-home residents cannot get out to shop for any of these things.

What more could you do for any shut-in to make him feel he is still a part of the outside world than to subscribe to his favorite newspaper? Or if he already gets a newspaper, then what about a subscription to a magazine he would enjoy receiving.

Someone recently subscribed to a newspaper for one of our women residents here. She was as joyous as a little child at Christmas over the gift and shared it with many others.

Other gifts can also lift our spirits and enhance our lives. My aide friends tell me that all nursing-home residents seem happiest with gifts of the kinds of toiletries they enjoyed before moving from their former homes. These gifts would include lotions, body powder, toothpaste or denture powder, perfumes, deodorants, mouthwash, and underarm antiperspirants.

Some like to have nail polish and polish remover.

Men like to receive blades for their razors. Or you might check their electric razors for them. I had the unhappy experience of a neighbor's faulty electric razor putting my TV out of business for one hour every day!

And, speaking of grooming, every nursing-home resident should have his own comb, hairbrush, and toothbrush. (Yes, believe it or not, every nursing home has patients who have forgotten to bring those necessary items.) They should have emery boards or files for filing their nails, daytime hair nets for some, sleeping nets for others. They should have needles, pins, and thread in their rooms. Nothing takes away a well-groomed appearance so quickly as a missing button! We have many of these items for sale in the secretary's office. Larger nursing homes usually have well-stocked shops. A small gift, but a big help to the one whose button is missing!

It is also most important for someone to check on the batteries in your loved ones' hearing aids if they are not able to order their own or the head nurse has not had time to test them.

One frequent visitor to Valley brings bird-seed for those of us who have feeders for wild birds. My nephew David brings me bushels of whole-ear corn. Another visitor reads aloud to those whose eyesight has waned. Some people bring books, quotations, tracts, and magazines to read, and sometimes clippings from newspapers or even cartoons. They are all appreciated as expressions of your loving concern.

Others come to do a bit of hand sewing from time to time. Putting in a hem or adding a button is sometimes difficult for arthritic fingers.

My friend Norma takes the time and energy to send me greeting cards for the many holidays throughout the year. She also brings me flowers from Sunday church services, baskets of fruit at Thanksgiving time, poinsettias at Christmas, and lilies at Easter. Best of all, she brings me her fetchin' pixie smile!

Many times my sister, Corrine, has brought something for my apartment. She always calls these little extras "housewarming gifts." One time it was a lovely, large folding screen that she had covered with a paisley-type design that matches the gold color in my carpet and walls.

My brother Lowell and his wife, Kay, keep me supplied with facial tissues and plain mint candies, specialties for the children who visit me. They also bring me unique stationery and napkins from their many short trips. Typical are bicentennial napkins from Kentucky, Marjorie Kinnan Rawlings' notepaper from Florida, and biblical cards from one of Ohio's Amish settlements.

Cassette tapes of interesting family happenings are most welcome. If the resident has a phonograph he'll appreciate records from time to time.

And after you finish this book you might also read *Green Winter: Celebrations of Old Age,* by Elise Maclay (*Reader's Digest* Press, 1977). Then you will know us better and know better what to do for us.

XVIII

Our Needs Are Simple

If I had known what trouble you were bearing . . .
What griefs were in the silence of your face . . .
I would have been more gentle and more
    caring . . .
And tried to give you gladness for a space . . .
I would have brought more warmth into the
    place . . .
If I had known.

—Mary Carolyn Davies

Not everything a person does for the nursing-home resident needs to be in the form of tangible gifts. Some downright unromantic, practical needs also need attention. One such concern is clothing.

Since Valley Home aides do our personal laundry, they ask that garments be of permanent-press, shrink-proof, and colorfast fabrics. Furthermore, all the aides agree that they unnecessarily waste hours dressing patients who are unable to dress themselves. For such patients, they urge you to buy all clothing larger than needed. It's important that sleeves be loose at the armholes and wrists.

If a patient is not entirely lucid, then it is vital for family members to take inventory of his wardrobe and general supplies and know when replacements are necessary. Mesh-knit, stretch-woven stockings are suggested for all patients. But no panty hose for those women who spend a lot of time in bed, especially if they are incontinent!

Then there is the problem of robes: choose long wraparound ones that open the entire way down the front, without zippers or buttons. Gowns should be long enough to be modest. Plunging necklines and sleeveless gowns are not good for very sick, older people whose circulation is often poor and who catch cold easily. Warm bed jackets are the answer for those who have already invested in their "pretty gowns." All underwear for those not completely ambulant comes under the larger sizes rule. Shoes should slip on easily if staff members are to perform efficiently.

I was surprised recently when one aide told me beds are a problem. Some are too high and some too low for the safety of the patient—another thing to check, if your loved one is at a nursing home where patients furnish their own beds.

Some ambulant patients, even those on walkers and in wheelchairs, if physically able, are delighted to have a short ride—within their own limits. No, you can't just come in and whisk somebody up and on you go. It takes time to prepare. Your guest needs to be warmly dressed. A nurse should be consulted first. You will need to arrange for aides to help you load and unload some individuals. Remember, every month, every year we live here, that outside world is changing fast. If possible, we would like to see it as it changes.

Corrinne ("Sis") and John have taken me to their home during summer vacation time. This means they have to have a local dealer bring to their home a size 122 breathing-oxygen tank. I have to take along my small portable E tank of breathing oxygen. I also need a wheelchair for shopping and sightseeing. I mention this because some residents' family members refuse to be bothered with even a walker, which is much less trouble. My trips take time and energy, but Sis and John realize the value of change to a nursing-home resident.

I'm also pleased and thankful that Myron and his wife, Jo, have been so willing to take me to the hospital, special doctors, and the like. I have felt actual pain when I have watched family members gruffly resist taking some of our residents to such places. How humiliated the resident must feel! The effort being made could so easily have been done cheerfully.

Beyond these uninspiring basics, our needs are really simple and not even terribly time-consuming. Most of them have to do with maintaining awareness and contact with the outside world.

When I visit a resident who is deaf, for example, I find it helpful to carry notepaper and pencil. Those who are deaf are likely to ask me questions, but they cannot hear my answers. I can pantomime some of the answers and use my head to motion "yes" or "no," but with the paper I am prepared to answer more complicated questions.

I don't suppose there is anything more difficult to adjust to than being removed from the atmosphere of a warm family home life. It's more than merely missing the presence of loved ones; it's the actual detachment from them.

I constantly worry about the health and welfare of my families. Without them life would be so empty for me. I wait eagerly to hear from them by mail and telephone and look forward to their visits in person.

Although many families find it difficult to share everything wholeheartedly with a relative who has entered a nursing home, it is possible to help a resident be aware of what's happening and continue to feel a part of the family circle.

Unexpected kindnesses have often buoyed my spirits, helped to pass my time joyfully, and given me courage to go on. I feel the most important of these kindnesses is the giving of self, an intangible quality most difficult to express in print. Momentary happinesses often bring lasting memories.

I am most grateful that in my younger days I faithfully visited friends and relatives in hospitals and nursing homes. But it never occurred to me that I could have done a lot more for people I didn't even know. I usually took a wee gift—flowers from our garden, a book, or a magazine. I am glad I did that much, but oh, I could do so much better now that I have lived here and observed!

Do you ever have a few spare moments between errands? If you are near a nursing home, why not run in a bit, if only for fifteen minutes, to say "Hi" to a resident? That is what Myron thought to do just this past week. He had half an hour between a stag breakfast and golf, so he spent it with me. I bubbled with appreciation!

There are many who want someone—anyone—to visit them just to have someone to talk to.

This reminds me of a conversation between a newly elected deacon and a senior deacon in my church. The new deacon remarked he just would not know what to talk about when he visited Jim or any other nursing-home patient. Our neophyte was told that all he had to do was to say, "Good morning, Jim. How are you?" Jim is the one who is hungry to talk, and he will take over from there.

It really is okay to let the residents do most of the talking if they seem so inclined. Usually their favorite subjects are their families, the homes they left, what they did when younger, and hobbies or travels they had. Many of the room-bound patients, especially, do not have the opportunity to join in actual conversations. Staff members just do not have time to sit down and talk.

I have often heard my late neighbor across the hall tell his dedicated pastor, "Now you keep quiet and let me do the talking. You get to talk all the time. Let me do the preaching this time!"

But when it's your turn to talk, giving honest compliments makes shut-ins feel confident and secure. Is their hair combed nicely? Tell them. Call them by their names. They get tired of being known only by their room numbers. Be sure you know their names before you enter their rooms. At Valley our names are on our entrance doors and we are called by our first names by the staff.

Mother loved her room here and was proud of her lovely antiques, both furniture and glass and china accessories.

Once in a great while, someone would visit her without saying anything about her pretties. After they left, she would comment, "They didn't say anything about my room." To tell the truth, they might just as well have stayed home as to omit that!

Why are some folks so parsimonious when it comes to compliments that could make others happy? Please remember this when you visit shut-ins. It gives them a lift and intensifies their interest in their immediate surroundings.

If the resident is well enough to have a telephone, for goodness' sake call ahead of time to find out when it is convenient to have company. Sometimes visitors have unintentionally done me more harm than good. Sometimes too many come on the same day. Perhaps they come just after I get back from our Valley Home Beauty Parlor, or right after the podiatrist has been working on my feet, or after or before a friend has taken me to a restaurant to eat. Result: a fatigued heart for me.

My favorite guests always courteously telephone ahead of time to see if it's convenient to visit. Then I can rest ahead of time and thoroughly enjoy their coming. I like to use my oxygen before my guests arrive. It takes extra oxygen to talk, you know.

When you telephone, you might like to ask if you can pick up something at the grocery, drug, or other stores. We don't mind asking for such favors if we know you are coming right by these places. We hesitate to ask you to retrace. Just try to imagine what it would be like for you to be shut in a nursing home with no means of personal transportation. Never forget that most of us are too proud to ask for favors.

Once you are in a patient's room, be sure to ask if there is anything you can do. If you see something that needs doing, do it. Of course, this will always depend on the capability of the resident.

Ask if you may open or close a window, sew on a button, reach for something high up in a closet, water the growing plants, write a letter, mail a letter, make a telephone call, pick up something from the floor, put fresh water in a bedside pitcher, put a shade up or down, pull draperies open or shut, take a note to the office, have prayer, read the Bible, tell jokes, start their clock or their watch, turn a light on or off, set the TV. If you turned it off when you came in, try to remember to turn it on again when you leave. It is a real help if you put chairs back where you found them, too.

Often some kind of an outing is a good idea, if weather and health permit it. One very dear new friend is the wife of one of the members of our board of trustees. I call her Merry Sunshine, the nickname her husband uses for her. She once took me on an inspiring short trek to the replica of an old Quaker

Meeting House, south of West Milton, Ohio. It was of special interest to both of us because her father and my husband's mother were both closely related to the late President Herbert Hoover, whose parents attended the original church.

There is another friend who volunteered to transport residents when Valley first opened. I was one of her first "passenger clients," but she rapidly changed from a mere transporter to a very dear friend. While she is young enough to be my daughter, we complement each other. Eleanor Whitesell is quite a family woman who baby-sits, helps me out when I'm sick, visits, and helps in the homes of her family. While deeply involved with church work, college classes, and an antique shop, she still has time for free-lance writing—and for me!

Some of the most delightful things we share are nature drives on remote country roads and in nearby parks. Laden with nature guidebooks and binoculars, we enjoy the water, birds, wild flowers, clouds, and trees. She insists I mention here that she gets as much pleasure out of our friendship as she gives, and is unaware of any generation gap. That makes Eleanor special to me!

But even if they cannot leave the nursing home, most wheelchair patients appreciate being pushed to another part of the building to visit a friend or, in some instances, outdoors on the walks.

Some people think, "That's what the nurse's aides and trained assistants are paid to do."

True. But every hospital and nursing home is understaffed. Besides, patients appreciate and enjoy tender loving care from someone dear to them. And don't forget how much joy it gives the giver, too!

It only takes a few minutes to cheer another person while visiting a relative. When Mary Jane Marker visits her mother, she stops in to see other people, too. She drops in long enough to bring her greetings and to leave a nosegay of flowers from her own garden.

A busy career woman with a husband, house, and family, Mary Jane still manages to visit often, bringing cheer to her own mother as well as to other residents. She even takes diet restrictions into consideration when she brings homemade cookies and candies to Valley residents.

My rainy-day girl, Margaret Andrew, has been a friend for many years. Why do I call Margaret my rainy-day girl? When I first came to Valley, she figured others would not come to see me on rainy days, so she came. Just a short visit from Margaret makes the sun shine in my life. She is sincere, learned, vivacious, and full of worthwhile ideas. And so full of projects! She shares them with me.

It may be a book she is writing, or collecting, organizing and donating the Darst family fine antique furniture to the Montgomery County Historical Society. Another time she may come with color slides or prints of her vacations or even just sit quietly smiling as I share my dreams with her.

"Sounds simple," I hear someone say. How long has it been since you did something that simple for someone in a nursing home? If you will do some of these helpful good deeds for those you know who are penned in nursing homes, they will love you for brightening their sometimes dreary lives.

Maybe the young man who wrote in a newspaper column was right when he said that we are helping to make "nonpersons" when we ignore our family and friends or treat them as if they have lived too long. He further said that if we would volunteer to help ease the loneliness found in long-term facilities, we would one day have, not just human warehouses where people sit alone waiting to die, but homes away from home where people *live*.

> If I had known what thoughts despairing drew you . . .
> Why do we never understand . . .
> I would have lent a little friendship to you . . .
> And slipped my hand within your lonely hand . . .
> And made your stay more pleasant in the land . . .
> If I had known.
> —Mary Carolyn Davies

APPENDIX I

Finding the Right Nursing Home—
The Search Begins

Most of the information available on nursing homes implies an immediate need, either because of a sudden illness or because of a chronic condition that worsens. One of the main points of this book is that everyone past middle age who might possibly need such a home someday should acquaint himself *now* with the various available facilities before he is suddenly forced into one. Not only will he be likely to find a better home, but adjustment will be much more pleasant.

What are the criteria you should use to evaluate nursing homes?

Obviously, a confirmed Christian will pray before and after visitations to be guided to the facility God wants him or his loved ones to have. We need to ask for wisdom and guidance in making decisions throughout life, of course. But when we are dealing with the fragile essence of aging, it is of the utmost importance to seek divine direction.

Many factors enter into the kind of residence you will select as best for you. Your age, the nature and condition of your illness, your finances, where the home is located, and whether you are single or married are key questions.

From my observations at Valley Home, I would not advise just one of a loving, companionable couple to move into a home permanently unless finances and health require it. I have witnessed some heartbreaking scenes here when good-byes had to be said.

The nursing home you choose depends largely on your physical and mental condition, as well as your doctor's prognosis and advice. A long-time bedfast patient should choose a skilled nursing home where comprehensive care can be given much as it is in a hospital. If you need little care, it might be better to select a retirement home or residential care center. The person who needs a bit more care might opt for an intermediate care facility (ICF). Many nursing homes provide a graduated plan of care from ambulant to bedfast.

There are both profit and nonprofit nursing homes. There are chain nursing homes just as there are chain grocery stores. One type of chain nursing home builds another link to better its service. The other type builds more to make more money. *Beware!*

Of all the problems of old age, finances are probably the most tragic. For most people the all-important deciding factor is economic. No longer do we equate the nursing home with the poorhouse. Poorhouse? Endowment payments in 1980 ranged anywhere from $20,000 to $60,000, plus a yearly service fee from $5,000 to $10,000. Since most people live in nursing homes for about two years, you can be proud to be financially able to afford it!

Most people will find it necessary to check their savings in all forms and the approximate value of their capital assets, as well as the coverage offered by the insurance they carry. (Many insurance policies cover skilled nursing homes only.) If this is your situation, your consideration of facilities may need to be limited to skilled nursing homes.

It's difficult to give figures, because costs vary widely, depending upon the community in which you live and the current status of the economy. The American Health Care Association says you can estimate your costs by learning the fees for a semi-private room in a local hospital. A semiprivate room in a nursing home runs from about twenty to thirty percent of the cost of comparable hospital care.

About sixty-five percent of nursing-home care in the United States is financed by state and federal medical aid under the umbrella of Social Security. An assistance program for needy and low-income persons, such aid is funded by federal and state taxes.

Since federal guidelines are broad, these assistance programs vary from one state to another. Generally, if a person's Social Security is not enough to meet the nursing-home costs, he can apply through Social Security for an SS-1. The SS-1 is a Social Security supplement.

If a person is eligible to participate in the medical aid program, he automatically receives both Medicare and state medical aid to cover the costs.

Another seven percent of American nursing-home costs is met by Medicare, a federal insurance program. To qualify for Medicare, you have to be over sixty-five, suffer from chronic kidney disease, or have been disabled for two years.

If you qualify for either of these assistance programs, you must be certain that the home you select is qualified. No payments are made to homes that are not eligible to participate in the medical aid programs. Some homes are even unwilling to accept aid payments. Your local Social Security office can give you detailed information about the restrictions on Medicare and medical aid recipients, as well as on the standards each nursing home must meet.

The remainder of nursing-home care is financed by pension funds, personal assets, Social Security, health insurance plans such as Blue Cross, veterans' benefits, and trade union or fraternal organizations.

Yet most of these programs need to be improved. Medicare and the various state aid programs need overhauling. There are organizations such as the Gray Panthers, the American Association of Retired Persons, and the National Retired Teachers' Association that are organizing to fight for better legislation to care for the aged.

Sufficient for this book is a plea to concerned

citizens to write their congressmen and the newly created Department of Health and Human Services to protest inadequacies. Fair legislation for the benefit of the aged is in everyone's best interest.

Equally important in considering economics is to check the financial status of the nursing homes you are considering. Recently, the precarious financial condition of a number of homes has been reported. What a tragedy to get nicely settled and have your home go bankrupt. If you have the ability to read financial records, ask the business manager of the homes you are considering to see them. Better still, have a person familiar with finance check them for you. It takes an exceptional person to interpret an institution's financial statement.

With all these considerations in mind, you'll be ready to begin your search. First ask your pastor, doctor, friends, and relatives for recommendations. Then phone your local Social Security office and the fire department for any information they might have about the nursing homes in the area.

Now with a large notebook to record your findings, start phoning nursing homes. Newspaper advertisements, telephone directory listings, and books on nursing homes will often provide the names and addresses of nursing and retirement homes in your area. Since state standards vary, if your state appears lax in supervision or too cold for your taste, you may want to consider a change in location or climate. This is usually unwise, though, if you have close ties to family, friends, or landmarks. For information about nursing homes in

other areas of the country, write:
The American Association for
Homes for the Aging
1050 17th Street, N.W. (Suite 770)
Washington, DC 20036
Telephone: 202-347-2000

You might also want to write to your denomina-
tional headquarters (and to those of other denominations with which you are comfortable) to request
information regarding church-related homes. It's a
good idea to enclose a large, self-addressed,
stamped envelope with your letter of inquiry.

By the time you've done this preliminary work,
your search has begun. Now that you know which
nursing homes you want to investigate, all you need
is the right questions to ask.

APPENDIX II

Finding the Right Nursing Home—
The Questions to Ask

It is wise to select as many homes for investigation as you have the time to visit. When you need a room, the home you've chosen may have no vacancies. There may be a waiting list. In order to be properly prepared, place your name on the waiting lists of at least two homes.

Once your visits have isolated several homes that seem promising, you will be ready to do further checking, again by telephone. If you are like most people, your first questions will be about finances. Often missed when checking costs are those hidden expenses. Request that the home send you any printed information it has, and then answer as many of the following questions as you can.

EXPENSES

Methods of Payment
1. Does this home accept Medicare or state medical aid payments?

2. Is there an entrance or endowment fee? How much is it? When is it payable? What is the refund policy?
3. Have this home's rates increased often, and how much?
4. Does cost vary according to square feet of floor space and other features of the room?

Doctors

1. Is there a staff doctor? What are the extra charges for his services?
2. Is your own family doctor or personal physician permitted to treat you?
3. Do podiatrists, dentists, optometrists, therapists, X-ray and laboratory technicians visit the home? What are the extra charges for their services? If they don't visit, are they near enough to be readily accessible?

Medicine

1. Can drugs be ordered from the pharmacy of your choice?
2. If the home orders the medicine from a doctor's prescription, are itemized bills provided?
3. Can you approve of orders from the drugstore prior to their purchase?
4. Is the family allowed to purchase over-the-counter items from "discount" stores rather than from delivering pharmacies?

Special Help

1. Is there an extra charge for any of the following:
   —serving trays in the room?
   —hand, tube, and intravenous feeding?

—care of the incontinent (catheters, colostomies, etc.)?
—hot pads?
—help in bathing and dressing?
—help in walking (use of wheelchairs, etc.)?

2. Is there a graduated fee according to the amount of care provided?
3. Does the home have a plan for transportation with reasonable charges?

Therapy

1. What mental, physical, and occupational therapy is included in the basic rates?
2. Are there extra charges for craft materials or the use of tools?

Equipment

Which of the following equipment carries an extra, hidden charge:

—Safety side rails?   —Hospital bed?
—Over-bed table?   —Bedside commode?
—Flotation cushions?   —Wheelchair?
—Geri-chair?   —Crutches?
—Walkers?   —Canes?
—Bedpans?   —Bed pads?
—Rubber pants?   —Catheters?
—Whirlpool?   —Oxygen?
—Syringes?
—Patient lift and springs?

Grooming

1. Are there beauty and barber shops in the building?
2. How often are they staffed?
3. What are the charges?

Special Diets
   1. Are special diets included in the basic rates? If not, how is the extra charge determined?
   2. Is there an extra charge for in-between-meal snacks if the doctor orders them?

Laundry
   1. What laundry services are available?
   2. Are linens and their laundry included in the basic rate?
   3. Is the resident permitted to use the home laundry facilities? If so, is there any extra charge?

Maintenance
   1. What types of minor repairs are made without charge?
   2. How much housekeeping is included in the basic rate?
   3. Are extra cleaning services available? What are the charges?
   4. Are residents permitted to hire outside help?
   5. Who furnishes light bulbs, toilet tissue, soaps, bath powder, rubbing lotions?

Once you have answers to these basic questions, you should be able to eliminate several homes from your list. Visit the ones that look like the best possibilities. Even a casual walk through a nursing home will reveal the answers to many of the points in my text.

LOCATION AND SURROUNDINGS

Location of Building
   Obviously, nursing homes should not be located too near any of the following:

—A lake or pool
—A river (because of the dangers of overflow or
   drowning)
—Landslides
—Railroad tracks
—A noisy, smoky factory
—Extra heavy traffic
—Buildings that are a fire hazard
—An airport
—Schools (occasionally the happy shouts of chil-
   dren can be enjoyable, but they can be very
   irritating when you are ill).

Outdoor Surroundings

1. Is there a safe entrance to the home grounds?
2. Are the premises well-kept?
   —Is the grass mowed?
   —Is the snow cleared?
   —Is the shrubbery trimmed and spaded?
   —Is there an absence of litter?
   —Can you see any garbage pails? (If you see
      them, they're in the wrong place, suggesting
      slovenly management and a lack of concern
      for hygiene.)
3. Are the walkways and driveways clean and in
   a good state of repair? Are they safe for walking
   and riding in wheelchairs?
4. Is adequate, convenient, safe parking provided at a distance not too far from the entrance to the building? (This is a convenience
   not only for residents but also for visitors.)
5. Is there a bus line near enough for family and
   friends who may need to take a bus?

FIRE AND SAFETY

I suggested in an earlier part of the book that you telephone the fire safety inspector at your local fire department. He can tell you which homes in your area have the highest safety ratings and how the homes on your lists meet the following safety specifications. Then when you visit, look for them yourself.

Fire Hydrants

1. How many fire hydrants are there?
2. In the case of a fire, are they near enough to the building?
3. Is the approach to the hydrants easily accessible?
4. Is the water volume adequate?

Fire Prevention

The building itself should be as fire resistant as possible. Throughout the building, look for the following:

1. Is there a modern sprinkler and alarm system? (The prohibitive cost of installing such systems in old buildings has caused some homes to close.)
2. Are there separating hall doors? Do they close automatically with the activation of the sprinkler system?
3. Is there an adequate number of portable fire extinguishers or standpipes throughout the building? Are they in plain view, with well-marked instructions for use?
4. Are there well-marked and well-lighted exits?
5. If this is a multistoried building, are there fire

escapes with enclosed staircases? Are there enclosed fire- and smoke-resistant, indoor staircases?

6. Are all doors wide enough (at least forty inches wide) to get hospital beds, stretchers and wheelchairs through?
7. Are paints and combustible cleaning fluids safely stored?
8. Are there definite smoking regulations? If "No Smoking" signs are used, are they in clear view?
9. Does the local fire department assist with a sufficient number of fire drills? ("Fire drills" in a nursing home do not involve emptying the building. But all staff need to know exactly where to be and which residents to help in the event of a fire.)

For more detailed information, write for a paperback, "Life Safety Code," to the National Fire Protection Association, 60 Batterymarch Street, Boston, MA 02110.

THE BUILDING

Building Entrance
1. Does the home you are visiting have entrance steps? (It shouldn't.) If so, are the steps easily negotiated? Is there outdoor carpeting, for example?
2. Is there a ramp? (A ramp is a splendid solution for outdated buildings with steps or even for new structures that for some reason could not have a ground level entrance.)

167

3. Do you enter on the ground level? (A ground-level entrance is the best of all entrances for the handicapped, as well as for everyone else.)
4. Is the entrance well lighted?
5. Does it say or imply "Welcome"?

The Lobby

The lobby gives everyone who enters his first impression of the building, so it should be inviting.

1. Is it well lighted?
2. Is it large enough?
3. Are the furnishings sturdy and in good taste?
4. Are the residents who are in the lobby well groomed?
5. Is the atmosphere cheerful? Boisterous or just friendly?
6. Does the lobby give you a good impression of the home?
7. Does it have a pleasant smell?

Hallways

Hallways are important to visitors as well as residents.

1. Are there skid-resistant floor surfaces throughout?
2. Are there handrails on both sides of the hall?
3. Are the halls well lit both day and night?
4. Are there well-marked exits?
5. Are portable fire extinguishers easily available? Do they have well-marked directions for their use?
6. Are the doorsills level with the rest of the flooring? (All floors from one end of the building to the other should be on the same level to

prevent falls and to accommodate the handicapped.)
7. Are service carts, wheelchairs, electrical cords,
cleaning apparatus, and packages out of sight?

THE KITCHEN

As far as your health is concerned, the kitchen is one
of the most critical areas in a nursing home. The
average person will not be able to properly assess
the quality and safety of the giant new kitchen
equipment. Conducted tours that let you compare
kitchens are helpful. One glance can tell you a great
deal. Try to see the kitchen when no one is working
in it as well as when it is in use.

Cleanliness
1. Is the kitchen crowded? (This causes food
spillage and hinders efficiency.)
2. Are counter tops free from soil from the last
meal?
3. Are floors mopped daily? (They should show
no dirt.)
4. Are dishes, silver, and utensils sterilized after
each meal?
5. Is the area around the refrigerator clean?
6. Is leftover food discarded after a short time?
7. Are kitchen staff members well groomed? Do
they have fresh uniforms daily?
8. Is the long hair of kitchen staff tied back or
coiffed?
9. Are their hands clean and well manicured,
with no long nails that may harbor bacteria?
10. Are kitchen noises kept to a minimum?

THE DINING ROOM

A communal dining room for all residents seems to meet the greatest approval. A good time for guests to visit the dining room is at mealtime. The most satisfactory way to check on the kitchen and dining room is to eat some meals there.

1. Is the dining room in a good, central location?
2. Is it adequate in size to prevent the crowding of chairs?
3. Is there accessibility by wheelchair and elevator?
4. Is there satisfactory lighting, both natural and artificial?
5. Is there a cheerful, pleasant atmosphere?
6. What attempt has been made to beautify the entire dining room and individual tables?
7. Is the furniture comfortable and attractive?
8. Are seats grouped into small clusters? Has an attempt been made to seat residents compatibly? Are seating assignments changed occasionally? Or do the residents sit wherever they wish at every meal?
9. Is help given to seat handicapped patients?
10. Is socializing encouraged?
11. Is the dining room clean? Are table mats large enough to protect place settings hygienically?
12. Are tabletops washed in a sanitary way?

ARTS AND CRAFTS ROOMS

Arts and crafts rooms are the most likely part of a nursing home to catch fire because they contain highly combustible materials. Good housekeeping in this area is essential. The room should be cleaned up at the end of each day.

1. Are paper, yarn, clippings, and shavings safely stored or disposed of properly?
2. Are paints and other painting materials, such as brush cleaners, carefully stored?
3. Are all tools (scissors, saws, knives, hammers) stored out of reach?
4. Are all electrical tools disconnected if they are not in use?
5. Are storage boxes off the floor to prevent accidents?
6. If there is a ceramics kiln, does it have a safety valve for heat control?
7. Is the door to the room locked when no supervisor is on duty?
8. Are fire and safety rules observed?

THERAPY ROOM

1. Do the fire and safety rules seem to be observed in the therapy room?
2. How does the therapy equipment compare to that of other homes?
3. Does the nursing home have the equipment you'll need?

AUDITORIUM

1. Are the aisles wide enough for wheelchairs?
2. Are the floors level, not elevated?
3. Is the room well ventilated? (Air conditioning is preferable if good judgment is used in keep-

ing temperatures moderate and consistent.)

4. Are there plainly marked, electrically lighted exit signs over the front and rear doors?

RESIDENTS' ROOMS

The information you can find for yourself about residents' rooms can be of great value to you in evaluating a nursing home. Visit as many as you can. What do you like about them? What disturbs you? (Sometimes nursing-home residents are reluctant to expose unpleasant facts, and members of the staff are understandably not likely to point out weak areas.)

First check the location of individual rooms in relation to the entrance, the business office, the nurses' station, the dining room, the auditorium, and the arts and crafts center.

Furnishings

1. Does the resident supply the furniture in each room, or is it supplied by the home?
2. How many accessories are permitted?
3. Are there TV outlets? Is there a communal aerial?
4. What other electrical appliances are permitted?
5. Are there enough convenient outlets?
6. If the rooms are not centrally air-conditioned, are there sleeves already installed for an air conditioner?
7. Are there access lines with plug-ins for telephones in the residents' rooms? Are regular telephone rates charged? Can a lock be placed on residents' telephones to prevent unau-

thorized phone calls?

8. Who furnishes draperies and shades?

MISCELLANEOUS

1. Are the residents' names on their doors?
2. Are safety rules posted in all rooms?
3. Are the rooms well lighted?
4. Are the rooms easy to heat?
5. Can surfaces be easily cleaned?
6. Is there a private bath?
7. Is it possible to lock the entrance door to the room for privacy?
8. Do you want a roommate? If so, how careful does this home seem to be in choosing a compatible one?
9. Is there any permanent objectionable odor in the rooms or adjoining hallways? (The lack of unpleasant odors suggests good care. Unpleasant odors suggest further investigation and questioning.)
10. How are residents' valuables protected?
11. Is there a call-bell system to the nurses' station in case assistance is needed?

BATHROOMS

Ask the following questions whether or not private bathrooms are available.

1. Are the bathroom floors skid-resistant?
2. Is the temperature of the water controlled to prevent scalding?
3. Does the bathroom have emergency buttons?

4. Are throw rugs prohibited?
5. Are there handrailings near the bathtub and commode?
6. Are the electric light switches at safe distances from the tub and shower?
7. Can a wheelchair be gotten into the bathroom?

CONVENIENCES FOR THE HANDICAPPED

1. Are there a sufficient number of the following and are they at proper heights for wheelchair patients and other handicapped persons?

—Drinking fountains	—Tables
—Telephone	—Windows
—Commodes	—Elevator controls
—Washbowls	—Curb ramps

2. Is there a safe, fenced-in outdoor area near the nursing home for patients?
3. Are there raised letters or figures for the benefit of blind and legally blind residents installed at each resident's doorway 4'6'' to 5'6'' above the floor?*
4. Are there knurled doorknobs or handles for all doorways that lead to hazardous areas?*

SOCIAL AND RELIGIOUS
PROVISIONS, PRACTICE, AND POLICY

Visitors

1. Are there limits as to when visitors may come and how long they may stay?
2. Are children welcome as visitors?
3. If this is a church home, is a resident's own pastor welcome to visit if he is of a different

denomination?

4. Does any organized volunteer group talk and read to residents, write letters, mend, and take ambulant residents shopping or riding?

5. Does the home discriminate on the basis of race, color, or creed?

Religion

1. Are ministers of different denominations from the sponsoring church allowed to hold services in lounges and other areas?

2. Does the home provide
   —church services   —social get-togethers
   —good music   —variety programs
   —lectures   —discussion groups
   —motion pictures   —prayer groups
   —Bible study   —freedom of religion

3. Are there any religious policies or practices with which you would be unhappy?

THE STAFF

The staff is of the utmost importance in evaluating a nursing home. Without a good staff, everything we have discussed is of little value. Do the faces of staff members reflect a genuine love for humanity, a desire to serve others, and other Christlike characteristics? Nursing and associated health careers demand a lot of the individual, and often it is only a commitment to Christian principles that prevents staff members from too easily giving way to impatience, irritation, and discourtesy.

Check the administrator's license date. It should be hanging in full view in his office. At the same time check the home's accreditation at your local Social Security office.

1. Is the home adequately staffed? (The recommended ratio is at least one staff member for every two residents.)
2. Do staff members meet state and federal requirements? (This information can be obtained through most local Social Security offices.)
3. Are members of the staff friendly, cooperative, quiet, well trained, pleasingly groomed, and professional?
4. Do the administrator and staff members seem to get along? Do staff members get along with each other?

Buildings are like people. They have personalities. The outer personality is easily visible. The inner personality is easily felt. After all your searching and study, does the building you are considering have a personality you can live with happily?

When you have answered questions like these for yourself and done this kind of research, I believe that you will find nursing homes one of the best solutions to the needs the aged have for adequate care. Gone will be any feeling of guilt about taking Grandma or Aunt Ella to a nursing home because you will have included her in the preparation!

One thing is sure: there no longer has to be a stigma to living in a nursing home. The answer lies in the selection of a satisfactory facility geared to the applicant. You can accomplish this only through intelligent advance planning and preparation.

I have lived at a nursing home since 1971 and I am not only content but satisfied with my choice. I'm especially glad I studied several nursing homes before I actually moved into one.

*Federal regulations. American National Standards Institute (ANSI).

Appendix III

Sample Application for Admission to a Nursing Home

Date: _____

1. Name of Applicant: _____

   Street Address: _____ City: _____

   Date of Birth—Month: _____ Day: _____ Year: _____ Age: _____

   Social Security Number: _____

   Marital Status—Married: _____ Single: _____ Widowed: _____

   Name of Husband or Wife: _____

   Address: _____

   If not living, date of death: _____

2. Names and addresses of children:

   1. _____
   2. _____
   3. _____
   4. _____
   5. _____

3. Church Membership:

   What is your church affiliation? _____

   Where do you worship at present? _____

   Name of Pastor: _____

   Address: _____

4. Reasons for wanting to enter this home: _____

   _____
   _____
   _____
   _____

5. Past and present occupation: _____

_____

6. Physical condition of applicant:

Eyesight? _____ Hearing? _____

Do you use crutches or a cane in walking? ____Wheelchair? _____

General condition? _____

State what, if any, serious illnesses you have had within the last five years:

_____

Physician who has attended you:

Name: _____

Address: _____

Date: _____

Do you use or take any special medication? _____

_____

_____

Do you use tobacco, alcohol, or narcotics in any form? Yes ___ No ___

If yes, explain: _____

Are you able to care for your own personal needs? _____

Do you require any special attention? _____

If so, explain fully: _____

_____

_____

7. List your present and previous interests:

Social—

Church: _____

School: _____

Clubs: _____

Hobbies and Crafts: Check those that interest you most—

☐ MUSIC ☐ TELEVISION ☐ GARDENING ☐ GAMES

☐ READING ☐ SEWING ☐ FLOWERS ☐ HANDWORK

☐ RADIO ☐ COOKING ☐ WOODWORKING ☐ PAINTING

8. Personal References: Give the names and addresses of three persons not related to you that you have known for a number of years:

	NAME	ADDRESS
1.	_____	_____
2.	_____	_____
3.	_____	_____

9. Have you ever been a resident in any other home or institution? _____
   If so, give name: _____

10. Where are you living now and under what arrangements? _____
    _____
    _____

11. How long can this arrangement continue? _____

12. When would you like to enter the home? _____

13. What type of accommodations would you like—
    Single room? _____ Double room? _____ Apartment suite? _____

14. Who should be notified in the event of your serious illness or death?

    NAME   ADDRESS   TELEPHONE NO.

    _____
    _____
    _____
    _____

15. Burial arrangements:
    Do you have a cemetery lot or right of interment? _____
    Holder of Deed _____
    Address _____
    Name of Funeral Home _____Phone _____
    Address _____

16. Financial Information *(This information is strictly confidential.)*
    A. *Real estate:* I own the following real estate in the county of
       _____ in the state of _____
       Description: _____.
       _____ Approximate market value $_____
       Do you have any interest, either legal or equitable, in any other property?
       Yes _____ No _____
       If so, explain: _____
    B. *Insurance:* I have health insurance with the following company:
       _____

    I have the following life insurance:

    COMPANY   AMOUNT   BENEFICIARY

    _____
    _____
    _____

    C. *Finances:* Please list below the financial resources and income that will
       finance your maintenance in the home:

APPENDIX III

Social Security $_____ per month Social Security Number _____

Pension $_____ per month_____ per year_____ Who pays it?_____

Annuity $_____ per month_____ per year_____ From what? _____

Other Income $_____ per month_____ per year_____ From what? _____

   D. *Personal property:* Cash assets:

      Savings account, bank and location _____

      _____ $_____

      Checking account, bank and location _____

      _____ $_____

      Stocks, bonds, notes, securities, mortgages, etc.:

COMPANY	NUMBER OF SHARES OR BONDS	
_____	_____	$_____
_____	_____	$_____

                    Total Cash and Securities $_____

   E. *Debts:*

      I have the following debts: _____

      _____

   F. *Signature of person or persons responsible for paying your financial obligations:*

      _____

17. To the best of my knowledge the above statements and information are true and correct as of this date.

    Date _____ Signed _____

PASTOR'S RECOMMENDATION

TO BE FILLED OUT BY THE APPLICANT:

Name of applicant _____

Present address _____ Phone _____

List the last three churches where you have been a member:

Church name	City
_____	_____
_____	_____
_____	_____

Church where membership is currently held: _____

Address: _____

Offices and/or positions held in the above-named churches

Position	Length of service	Church
_____	_____	_____
_____	_____	_____
_____	_____	_____
_____	_____	_____

Date and place of conversion_____ _____
Date and place of baptism_____ _____

TO BE FILLED OUT BY THE PASTOR:

What additions or corrections, if any, would you make to the above statements?
_____
_____

Is the applicant presently a member of your church? _____
How long have you known the applicant? _____
The applicant's church attendance has been:
☐ Regular   ☐ Occasional   ☐ Rare
Briefly describe the character of the applicant: _____
_____
_____

Additional pertinent information: _____
_____

Date: _____ Pastor's Name: _____
Address: _____

MEDICAL HISTORY

To be filled out by the resident and/or physician
Must be received before the resident will be admitted

Name: _____
Last   First   Middle
Date of birth: _____ Sex: _____ Race: _____

I. Childhood diseases:	Yes	No	Don't remember
Chicken pox	☐	☐	☐
Mumps	☐	☐	☐
Measles	☐	☐	☐

II. Adult difficulties:	Yes	No	Date
Diabetes	☐	☐	_____

183

APPENDIX III

Tuberculosis	☐	☐	_____
Heart trouble	☐	☐	_____
Mental illness	☐	☐	_____
Epilepsy	☐	☐	_____
Pneumonia	☐	☐	_____
Glaucoma	☐	☐	_____
Cataracts	☐	☐	_____

III. Hospitalizations:

Date	Cause	Length of Stay
_____	_____	_____
_____	_____	_____
_____	_____	_____
_____	_____	_____

IV. Broken Bones:

Date	Location of break
_____	_____
_____	_____

V. General questions:

Do you have any known drug sensitivities? ☐ No ☐ Yes

If yes, list them: _____

Known allergies? ☐ No ☐ Yes If yes, list them: _____

Do you wear a hearing aid? ☐ No ☐ Yes How Long? _____

Do you wear glasses? ☐ No ☐ Yes How Long? _____

When did you last have your eyes checked? _____

Do you wear dentures? ☐ No ☐ Yes

When were you last checked by a dentist? _____

Do you walk without assistance? ☐ No ☐ Yes

If no, what do you use:

☐ cane   ☐ walker   ☐ crutches   ☐ wheelchair

_____ _____
Name of person (if other than resident) filling out form   Date

_____ _____
Physician   Date

PHYSICIAN'S EXAMINATION

Name _____

Age _____ Weight _____ Height _____

Blood pressure _____

184

Did you find any abnormalities of the following? If so, explain under "Remarks."

Skin_____ Thyroid_____ Throat_____ Teeth_____ Nose_____ Eyes_____

Ears_____ Breast_____ Uterus_____ Heart_____ Blood vessels_____

Lungs_____ Stomach_____ Intestines_____ Liver_____ Kidneys_____

Spine_____ Extremities_____ Nervous system_____ Pancreas_____

Bladder_____ Prostate_____ Gall bladder_____ Pulse_____

Report of chest X-ray or T.B. skin test (must have been taken within the last twelve months).

_____

Diagnosis:

Primary _____

_____

Secondary _____

_____

If patient has cancer, state location. _____

Extent: _____

Type of treatment given: _____

Prognosis _____

_____

Medication (use back if necessary):

List all medications:	Dosage	Frequency
_____	_____	_____
_____	_____	_____
_____	_____	_____
_____	_____	_____
_____	_____	_____
_____	_____	_____
_____	_____	_____
_____	_____	_____
_____	_____	_____

Allergies _____

Diet: ☐ regular ☐ special Type: _____

Remarks: _____

_____

_____

APPENDIX III

I hereby declare that I have been acquainted with the above named applicant for
_____ and have this _____ day of _____ 19_____ examined
him or her, and I certify that the answers to the above questions are true.

_____
(Signature of Physician)

_____
(Address)

Appendix IV

Sample Letter
from a Nursing Home

Dear resident of Valley Home:

With the approach of 1977 the Board of Trustees considered many items in order to delay an increase in monthly service charges. We wish to call to your attention a number of decisions and remind you of our policies included in each of your admission contracts as resident obligations.

Valley Home does not furnish linens, towels, blankets, or personal furnishings for its residents but permits each resident to bring with him his own belongings. Bath towels, washcloths, sheets, pillow cases, etc., when washed as needed, wear out and must be replaced. It is requested that each resident (or responsible party) check to insure that a sufficient quantity of these items, in good condition, is available and properly marked for his use.

APPENDIX IV

The Board of Trustees has adopted the following rental rates to be charged residents for equipment needed after January 1, 1977:

	Monthly Rental
Hospital Bed with Rails	$20.00
Safety Side Rails	4.00
Wheelchairs	10.00
Flotation Cushions	3.00
Bedside Commode	4.00
Patient Mobile Chair	10.00
Patient Lift & Slings	12.00
Overbed Table	2.00
Walkers	3.00

A problem has also been prevalent as to late payment of service charges. Therefore, effective January 1, 1977, a late charge of $10.00 will be added to each monthly invoice not paid by the tenth of the month.

Payment for all medication is the responsibility of the resident; therefore Valley Home will no longer supply without charge nonprescription drugs and medical supplies from stock. For those items furnished at cost, a pharmacy charge will be added to the monthly statement.

State law prohibits the use of plastic wastebaskets in resident rooms. Therefore it is requested that those residents now using plastic wastebaskets remove them from their rooms and replace them with metal wastebaskets.

Valley Home permits those residents physically capable of doing their personal laundry to use the small Maytag washer in our laundry room without charge. The commercial washer (Westinghouse) is not to be used by the residents. Residents are to furnish their own laundry detergent, bleach, and fabric softeners.

Housekeeping service is furnished for each resident's room on a weekly schedule; daily requests for maid service cannot be granted. All requests for maintenance and additional housekeeping must be made through the office.

Food costs continue to increase, but our guest meal charges will remain unchanged: breakfast, $1.00; noon meal, $1.50; and evening meal, $1.25. Payment for guest meals should be made to the office or may be charged and placed on your monthly statement.

Thank you for your cooperation in our effort to keep down the cost of operations here at Valley Home.

Sincerely,

John Jones
Administrator

BIBLIOGRAPHY AND SUGGESTED READING

BOOKS

Burger, Sarah G. and D'erasmo, Martha. *Living in a Nursing Home.* New York: Seabury Press, 1976.

Curtin, Sharon R. *Nobody Ever Died of Old Age.* Boston: Little, Brown and Company, 1973.

Faunce, Frances Avery. *The Nursing Home Visitor.* Nashville: Abingdon Press, 1969.

Hooker, Susan. *Caring for Elderly People.* Boston: Routeledge and Kegan Paul, Ltd., 1976.

Horn, Linda, and Griesel, Elma. *Nursing Homes.* Boston: Beacon Press, 1977. (This book is an expose, but it suggests many remedies and really should rank as a textbook. The authors and Maggie Kuhn, who wrote the introduction, are Gray Panther-oriented.)

Life Safety Code. Boston: National Fire Protection Association, n.d.

Maclay, Elise. *Green Winter: Celebrations of Old Age.* New York: Reader's Digest Press, 1977.

Nassau, Jean Baron. *Choosing a Nursing Home.* New York: Thomas Y. Crowell, 1973.

PAMPHLETS ON AGING

The following pamphlets are available free of charge. When requesting copies, enclose a stamped, self-addressed business envelope.

A Brief Explanation of Medicare. U.S. Department of Health, Education and Welfare, Social Security Administration, HEW Publication No. (SSA) 76-10043, U.S. Government Printing Office, Washington, DC 20402.

Hearing Aids Selected: 1976. Department of Medicine and Surgery, Veterans Administration, Washington, DC 20402.

Hearing Loss. DHEW Publication No. (NIH) 73-157, Superintendent of Documents, U.S. Government Printing Office, Washington, DC 20402.

It Can't Be Home. Superintendent of Documents, U.S. Government Printing Office, Washington, DC 20402.

Let's End Isolation. Administrator on Aging, Office of Human Development, Publication OHD75-20129, HEW, Washington, DC 20201.

Medicaid and Medicare: Which Is Which? Consumer Information Center, Pueblo Memorial Airport, Pueblo, CO 81009.

Nursing Home Care. U.S. Department of Health, Education and Welfare, Social and Rehabilitation Service, Medical Services Administration, Washington, DC 20201.

Thinking About a Nursing Home: American Health Care Association, 1200 15th Street, N.W., Washington, DC 20005.

Your Medicare Handbook. U.S. Department of Health, Education and Welfare, U.S. Government Printing Office, Washington, DC 20402.

Acknowledgments

To my friends and acquaintances for their sincere interest and deep faith, which encouraged me with my project—even to the one staff member whose cynical attitude made me all the more determined that I could write a book even though I was over eighty!

To newspaper columnists Glee Krentz, Jean Kappell and Ed Kemper for the boosts they gave my book and my morale.

To my senior pastor, Dr. William Schram, who gave me my biggest lift of all in words of real encouragement.

To my doctor, Austin Hammond, M.D., and his wife, Marian, a registered nurse, and the other nurses at Valley for the wisdom they displayed in not only letting me write but encouraging me to continue writing within my limitations.

To Valley's administrator, Joseph Lefkovitz, for his continuing encouragement, his understanding of my health problems, and much helpful information.

To the cooperative nurse's aides who gave me suggestions.

To my sister, Corrinne Hutchins Hock, and to Norma Goodman, a member of the board of deacons from Westminster Church, who helped me with editing as the manuscript developed.

To my sister's husband, John Hock, who did hours of tiresome errand work for me I could not do for myself: purchasing stationery and making trips to the photocopier and post office.

To the many who helped me with typing, especially my dear friend Sue, who laboriously and perfectly typed and retyped what seemed to me like a never-ending number of pages. Her contribution to this book is inestimable. She was always available for consultation about the manuscript. Since I am physically unable to do the work myself, she did it for me. She patiently interpreted some almost illegible manuscripts and saved me hours of copying.

And, finally, to the Dayton-Montgomery County Public Library staff who gave me the extra help without which I could not have written this book. The assistance I received by telephone from the literature department was invaluable. Dave Roach and Leon Bey of the bookmobile department and all the department's helpers took so much interest, anyone could have thought this was their book.